SHAKING UP PARKINSON DISEASE

FIGHTING LIKE A TIGER, THINKING LIKE A FOX

A Book for the Puzzled, the Hopeful, the Willing, and the Prepared

by

ABRAHAM LIEBERMAN M.D.
NATIONAL MEDICAL DIRECTOR
NATIONAL PARKINSON FOUNDATION INC.

JONES AND BARTLETT PUBLISHERS
Sudbury, Massachusetts
BOSTON TORONTO LONDON SINGAPORE

This book was made possible through a grant to the National Parkinson Foundation, Inc. from Novartis Pharmaceuticals Corporation

World Headquarters
Jones and Bartlett Publishers
40 Tall Pine Drive, Sudbury, MA 01776
978-443-5000
info@jbpub.com
www.jbpub.com

Jones and Bartlett Publishers Canada
2406 Nikanna Road Mississauga, ON
L5C 2W6
CANADA

Jones and Bartlett Publishers International
Barb House, Barb Mews
London W6 7PA
UK

Production Credits
Sponsoring Editor: Christopher Davis
Editorial Assistant: Thomas Prindle
Production Editor: Anne Spencer
Manufacturing Buyer: Therese Bräuer
Text and Cover Design: Anne Spencer
Production Services: Nesbitt Graphics, Inc.
Printing and Binding: Malloy Lithography
Cover Printing: Jaguar Advanced Graphics

Library of Congress Cataloging-in-Publication Data
Lieberman, A. N. (Abraham N.), 1938-
Shaking up Parkinson disease: fighting like a tiger, thinking like a fox / by Abraham Lieberman.
p. cm.
ISBN 0-7637-1866-1
1. Parkinson's disease-Popular works. I. Title: Shaking up Parkinson disease.
II. Title.
RC382 .L544 2001
616.8'33-dc21
2001025721

Printed in the United States
05 04 03 02 01 10 9 8 7 6 5 4 3 2 1

Preface

Each day, every day, people with Parkinson disease (PD) awaken, trapped in their bodies. They move slowly, their limbs are stiff, their hands shake, and their legs won't do what they want them to. They shuffle instead of taking long strides, and periodically "freeze," unable to move. Picture being in a car and the car won't start when you turn the key. Or after it starts, the brake, not the accelerator, kicks in. You can't leave the car — because the car is you. And if someone, a doctor, jump-starts you with a drug, you'll do well — for a while — and then you're stuck again. You talk to your family, your friends, to other people with Parkinson. You exercise, you change your diet, you meditate, and everything works again. Later, you add another drug. You grow closer to your family, your friends — and your feelings. And you pray — yes you pray. For as important as science is, belief is equally important.

Who Gets Parkinson Disease?

This book explains PD: its main symptoms of rigidity, tremor, slowness of movement, and difficulty with balance. It shows where in the brain PD starts, its anatomy and chemistry. It explains why people with PD have difficulty walking, speaking, and writing. It points out that PD, contrary to what you think, is not just a disease for old people, for your grandmother or grandfather. Parkinson is also a disease for young people, hitting and bewildering them as they start their careers, their families, their lives.

Parkinson is often thought of as a disease of famous people; most would trade fame for a cure. These famous people, both living and dead, have been diagnosed with PD: Muhammad Ali, Salvador Dali, Michael J. Fox, Francisco Franco, Adolf Hitler, Pope John Paul II, and Morris Udall. Why? The book speculates on the association.

How Parkinson Works

The book explains how PD advances, it explains the stages of PD, and explains how you can best live within them. The book explains the autonomic nervous system, the "secret" part of the brain without which we could not live. It explains how in PD the autonomic nervous system affects your breathing, your swallowing, and your bowel movements. It explains how the autonomic nervous system affects your sex life. And it explains what you and your spouse can do about a faulty autonomic nervous system.

The book discusses the physical pain of PD, another "secret" of PD, except to those of you who hurt and are told, "it's only in your head."

The Emotional Toll of Parkinson

The book discusses anxiety and depression in PD. Forty percent of people with PD are anxious, and forty percent are depressed, and many are anxious and depressed. The book explains how you can measure anxiety or depression and determine if it is reasonable or unreasonable, appropriate or inappropriate. By measuring anxiety and depression you'll understand them, be able to explain them to your family, your doctor, your minister, and eventually be able to master them.

Anxiety and depression in PD isn't only about physical disability. Some of you who are the least disabled are the most depressed, and some of you who are the most disabled, are the least depressed. Why? I address that here.

Difficulty sleeping in PD is related to immobility, anxiety, depression, and, in part, to the drugs for PD. The book explains how you can learn why you are having difficulty and correct it.

Parkinson affects thinking, another "secret" of PD, one seldom discussed for fear of frightening people. While the dementia of PD is not something to worry about in the beginning, it is a "ticking bomb" and, eventually, will affect 30% of PD sufferers; which is why research is so important; which is why the world must rid itself of PD as it rid itself of plague, small pox, and polio.

Is It Parkinson or Something Else?

The book discusses diseases confused with PD, including Essential Tremor, Multiple System Atrophy (or Shy Drager Disease), Progressive Supranuclear Palsy (abbreviated PSP), Restless Legs, and Dystonia. These are strange sounding, difficult to pronounce words until you are diagnosed with them and you seek to find the differences between them and PD. Is it better or worse to have one of them or PD?

The book discusses things known to cause PD: viruses, head injuries, drugs, heavy metals, and carbon monoxide. These account for less than 5% of all cases of PD; and, curiously, may not be PD. The precise cause of PD is unknown. It is more common as we grow old, it is less common among women, and it may be environmental or genetic. Could the Gulf War Syndrome lead to PD? Will the unraveling of the human genome lead to a cure? These scenarios are discussed in the book.

Treating Parkinson Disease

I have spent 35 years treating people with PD. My colleagues and I were among the first to test and develop drugs such as Sinemet, Comtan, Mirapex, Permax, Requip, and selegiline. The book provides insights into how PD drugs work, when a drug should be started, when it should be changed, and when it should be stopped, as well as surgery for PD: when it should be done, and who may benefit. The book discusses the importance of exercise to combat rigidity and immobility, of nutrition to promote good general health, of emotional support, and of a belief in a Greater Good — a Higher Power to keep you sane.

Much of the above is explained through the stories of eleven people with PD. These are "composite" people, several people the author has known and blended together. Each composite person becomes a real person because the stories are true. They are brought together through the National Parkinson Foundation (NPF) Quality of Life Examination, an examination that looks at all aspects of a PD person's life: mobility, activities of daily living, emotions, thinking, and bodily functions. The NPF Quality of Life Examination will enable you to measure your progress, or lack of it, help you understand where the problem may be, and enable you to discuss it with your doctor in terms both of you can understand and act on.

The stories include Anna, a 57-year-old woman who is diagnosed and followed for five years; Melvin, a 62-year-old state senator with PD who wants to run for governor; Jack Jr., a 60-year-old man whose father had PD and whose brother-in-law, Dan, has PD—so, of course Jack Jr. can't have PD, because it is "improbable;" Jerry, a 35-year-old dentist who, while having an affair, discovers he has PD, and, convinced he brought it on himself, searches for a cause; Martha, a 57-year-old woman who, "looking much younger than she is," is too vain to have PD; Lenny, a 60-year-old man with Shy Drager, a disease worse than PD, who finds through God the courage to help others; George, a 75-year-old genius who develops PD and dementia; Pete, who's struggling with PD until he learns how his drugs work; and Jill, a caregiver whose husband, father-in-law, and brother-in-law have PD.

This book contains insights, messages, and thoughts from celebrities who know PD. Christine Lahti, Holly Robinson Peete, and Senator Paul Wellstone speak about their parent's PD. Henny Backus and Norma Udall speak about their husbands' PD. Cliff Robertson speaks about his friend, Congressman Mo Udall's PD. And Jack Anderson and Earl Ubell speak about their PD.

People with PD and their families must understand it and approach it unlike anything they've faced in their life. Because, although you never wished for PD, or wanted it, it is there and it is part of your life. To live with it you'll have to fight it as fiercely, as ferociously, as persistently as a tiger. And you'll have to think about getting around it and outsmarting it as cunningly, as cleverly, as daringly as a fox.

If you know someone who has PD, buy two copies of the book, one for you and one for them. And if you have PD, buy two copies of the book, one for your bedside, and one for when you leave your house, because, like your credit card, you won't want to leave home without it.

About the Author

If you or a family member has Parkinson disease you will recognize Abraham Lieberman, MD as the National Medical Director of the National Parkinson Foundation, a Professor of Neurology at the University of Miami, and the Co-Director of the National Parkinson Foundation University of Miami Parkinson Disease Center.

Dr. Lieberman is an internationally recognized expert on Parkinson disease, the author or co-author of five books on Parkinson disease, has treated many famous people with Parkinson disease, and is an expert on Adolf Hitler's PD. His manual on PD has been printed and reprinted, translated into five languages (French, Italian, Spanish, Portuguese, and Russian), and, over 15 years, more than one million copies have been distributed, free of charge, world-wide. His interactive Web site, *www.parkinson.org,* containing updates on PD and answering questions about the disease, is viewed by 10,000 people daily.

Dr. Lieberman is a 1959 graduate of Cornell University, and a 1963 graduate of the New York University School of Medicine. He is board certified in neurology and psychiatry, and is a Fellow of the American Academy of Neurology, the American Neurological Association, and the Movement Disorder Society. He is licensed in Florida and California.

Dr. Lieberman trained in neurology at Bellevue Hospital in New York from 1964 to 1967. Bellevue is one of the largest and busiest city hospitals in the United States. Bellevue serves all the people in New York and has been a leader in the delivery of care and in the training of doctors. During the Vietnam War, Dr. Lieberman was a neurologist at the United States Air Force Hospital in Tachikawa, Japan, from 1967 to 1969.

Between 1969 and 1970, Dr. Lieberman did a fellowship in pharmacology at New York University under the direction of Dr. Menek Goldstein — one of the pioneers in understanding the biology and chemistry of the brain. Dr. Lieberman learned the theories and practicalities of Parkinson research, and it was through Dr. Goldstein that Dr. Lieberman met and came to know the great figures in Parkinson research.

Between 1970 and 1989, Dr. Lieberman climbed the academic ladder at New York University from instructor, to assistant professor, to associate professor, to professor of neurology. He was the principal or co-principal investigator of more than 200 grants and studies. These included studies on Alzheimer disease, brain tumors, coma, depression, epilepsy, migraine headaches, nerve and muscle disease, stroke and Parkinson disease, with more than 75% of the studies devoted to PD. Most of the studies involved inventing ways of evaluating these diseases, finding new ways of treating them, and explaining them to perplexed, worried, and puzzled patients. The studies were complemented by a large and varied neurology practice, seeing people from every corner of the globe who came to NYU. Here, Dr. Lieberman, working with world-renowned authorities in medicine, neurology, surgery, and psychiatry, came to appreciate the role of anxiety, fear, panic, and depression in every disease.

Beginning in 1970, and accelerating after 1980, Dr. Lieberman's practice centered on Parkinson disease. This intensified in the nine years at the Barrow Neurological Institute in Phoenix, Arizona, between 1989 and 1998. Here, Dr. Lieberman, with generous support from Muhammad and Lonnie Ali, the Barrow Neurological Institute, St. Joseph's Hospital, and the Phoenix community, started the Muhammad Ali Parkinson Research Center. The Center, located in central Phoenix, serves patients from every part of Arizona and the world — regardless of ability to pay.

Dr. Lieberman's interest in Parkinson disease was stimulated by a revolutionary breakthrough, the introduction of levodopa, L-dopa — by Dr. George Cotzias, in 1967. The interest was sharpened by the presence of gifted scientists in biochemistry, neuro-chemistry, neuro-pharmacology, neuro-physiology, and neuro-psychology at NYU. With colleagues at NYU, the Barrow Neurological Institute, and the University of Miami, Dr. Lieberman has authored or co-authored more than 200 articles on Parkinson disease and related diseases and published in major medical and neurology books and journals including: the New England Journal of Medicine, the Lancet, the Journal of the American Medical Association, the Annals of Internal Medicine, the Annals of Neurology, the Archives of Neurology, Neurology, the Journal of Neurology, Neurosurgery, Psychiatry, and the Journal of Pharmacology and Therapeutics.

First as Scientific Director of the American Parkinson Disease Association, and now as National Medical Director of the National Parkinson Foundation, Dr. Lieberman pioneered the education of people with Parkinson disease, their spouses, care-partners, family, and friends. In these endeavors he's been fully supported and encouraged by Mr. Nathan Slewett, the volunteer Chairman of the National Parkinson Foundation. In the past 35 years Dr. Lieberman has seen, examined, and counseled more than 35,000 people with Parkinson disease. This book is a distillation of that experience and learning.

On a personal note Dr. Lieberman has been married 35 years to Ina Lieberman, a pediatric anesthesiologist. They have four children, one daughter-in-law, one almost daughter-in-law, and three grandchildren. At age 6, Dr. Lieberman had polio, spending 18 months in hospitals, clinics, and rehabilitation centers. Dr. Lieberman knows adversity, anxiety, depression, fear, panic, and hope as a neurologist and as a patient.

Dedication

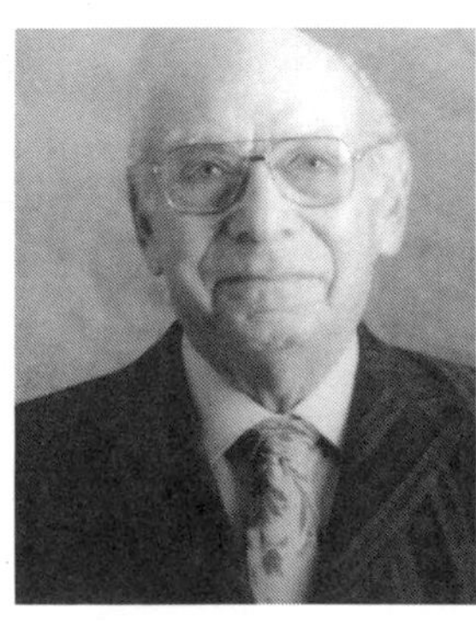

This book is dedicated to Nat Slewett, Chairman of the National Parkinson Foundation. At a time when people retire and enjoy the sweet fruit of their life's labors, Mr. Slewett took over the NPF. In 15 years he remade the NPF from a "store front clinic in Miami" into an eminently respected global organization. He established NPF Centers of Excellence providing care, research, education, and respite to hundreds of thousands of people with PD. NPF Centers of Excellence are found at major clinics and universities from Massachusetts to Miami, from Washington, DC, to Washington State, from Pennsylvania to California, from Argentina to British Columbia, from Beijing to Paris, and Tel Aviv to Tokyo.

He has, through friends, business associates, corporations, and private foundations raised nearly 75 million dollars for research in PD. And he has given generously not only of his time, but also of his own money. He has lobbied tirelessly in Washington, London, Austin, Tallahassee, and Sacramento — wherever there's a president, a prime minister, a governor, a senator, or a congressman, anyone who can unlock money for PD. As great as Nat's efforts are, it is the government that has the vast sums of money needed to cure PD.

He has spoken to large national audiences on television. He has spoken at seminars of research scientists. And, one on one, he has comforted people with PD. He has spoken at several meetings in a day in city after city for days on end never asking if he has the strength, knowing he will find the strength because he has the cause.

He has inspired doctors, research scientists, and people with PD. He has been and is a champion of everyone with PD. He takes no fees for speaking, he pays his own expenses, he receives no salary, he is a volunteer. And if we had another Nat Slewett we would not need this book, because PD would be a memory.

With Thanks

The insightful, inspired, and willing help of Ruth Hagestuen RN, Susan Imke RN, Kim Seidman, and Mary Willis is acknowledged with deep appreciation.

Table of Contents

CHAPTER

I

Parkinson: A Disease of Moving

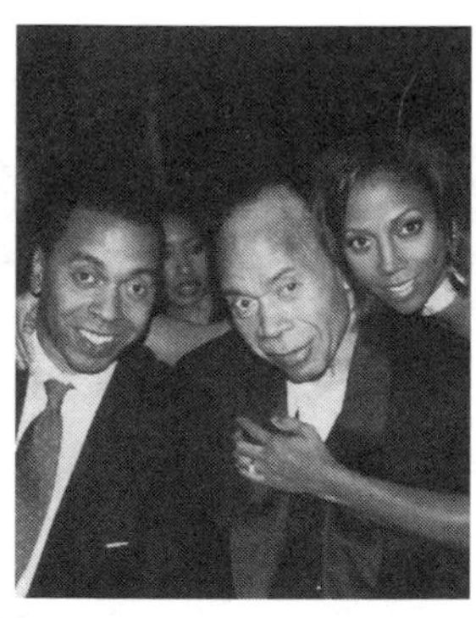

Holly Robinson Peete, Actress

"I was entering my freshman year of college and my father came to visit me. When he was leaving in the cab, he was walking with this funny limp in his knee. It was the strangest thing. He was a real joker and a comedy writer, so I remember saying to him, 'Hey Dad, why are you walking like Fred Sanford?' We joked about it, but when I came home three months later for Christmas he was diagnosed with Parkinson disease. It was the first time I ever heard the name Parkinson — that was before the information highway, before the Internet, before anything. I scoured every library that I could to find any piece of information on Parkinson, but there wasn't a lot of information. It was a very empty feeling. The only words I kept seeing were 'incurable' and 'neurological.' I was totally lost. There was nothing like this book when my father was diagnosed.

"There is much more knowledge today than there was twenty years ago. You'll find information that I never had access to. If you or a family member are diagnosed, become a scholar of it. There is so much you can do to fight the disease."

Parkinson disease (PD) is a slowly progressive disease of the brain. Although it mainly affects mobility, it can also affect emotions, thinking, communicating, and bodily functions (including those of the bowel and bladder). There are approximately 1.2 million people with PD in the United States and Canada, 3,500 people with PD for every one million people. The *incidence,* the number of new people diagnosed with PD each year, is approximately 60,000. Because the period between the onset of symptoms and diagnosis (latency) is between 2 and 5 years, it is estimated that for every person who is diagnosed with PD, there are at least two who have PD but have not been diagnosed.

The peak onset of PD is at age 60. PD affects 1% of all people aged 60 or older, and 2% of all people aged 70 or older. However, PD is not just a disease of middle or old age: 15% of PD patients are 50 years of age or younger, 10% are 40 or younger, and PD occurs in teenagers. PD affects men more than women: 55 men for every 45 women. PD affects Caucasians more than people of color. The disease progresses from minor to major disability over 10 to 25 years. There are effective treatments for PD.

Diagnosing Parkinson Disease

Parkinson disease is diagnosed based on the information given to the doctor and an examination performed in the doctor's office. Blood tests, urine tests, X-rays or tests such as magnetic resonance imaging (MRI) can be done to rule out conditions that mimic PD. In some people a response to levodopa, the principal drug used to treat PD, can confirm the diagnosis, as the diseases that mimic PD don't respond to levodopa.

The Quality of Life in Parkinson Disease

Parkinson disease affects mobility and this, in turn, may affect one's ability to perform ordinary daily activities. It is these aspects of PD that are measured and tested in the doctor's office. Less well known is that PD may also affect emotions, thinking, interpersonal relations, and certain body functions. In trying to measure the quality of life of people with PD, all of the above must be considered.

The following Quality of Life Scale represents an attempt to inform PD patients and their families how different aspects of PD influence quality of life, how the progression of PD affects it, and how different treatments and coping strategies can improve it.

QUALITY OF LIFE SCALE

Answer the following questions using the scoring system below.

Never:	score "0"	means you never had difficulty with this during the week
Some:	score "1"	means you had difficulty on 1, 2, or 3 days during the week
Often:	score "2"	means you had difficulty on 4, 5, 6, or 7 days during the week

Mobility

How often in the past week did you:

1.	Have difficulty turning in bed?	0	1	2
2.	Have difficulty getting up from a chair?	0	1	2
3.	Have difficulty carrying things?	0	1	2
4.	Have difficulty turning when walking?	0	1	2
5.	Freeze and become unable to walk?	0	1	2

6.	Have a noticeable tremor?	0	1	2
7.	Feel unsteady or wobbly?	0	1	2
8.	Have difficulty walking to the house?	0	1	2
9.	Have difficulty walking in public?	0	1	2
10.	Need someone to go outside with you?	0	1	2
11.	Skip something you wanted to do?	0	1	2
12.	Fall?	0	1	2

Activities of Daily Living

How often in the past week did you:

13.	Have difficulty going to the toilet?	0	1	2
14.	Have difficulty bathing or showering?	0	1	2
15.	Have difficulty shaving or applying make-up?	0	1	2
16.	Have difficulty dressing or undressing?	0	1	2
17.	Have difficulty writing legibly?	0	1	2
18.	Have difficulty feeding yourself?	0	1	2
19.	Have difficulty holding a cup or glass?	0	1	2
20.	Have difficulty swallowing?	0	1	2

Emotional State

How often in the past week did you:

21.	Feel depressed?	0	1	2
22.	Feel isolated or lonely?	0	1	2
23.	Feel sad or tearful?	0	1	2
24.	Feel angry or bitter?	0	1	2
25.	Feel anxious or tense?	0	1	2
26.	Worry about the future?	0	1	2
27.	Have difficulty sleeping?	0	1	2
28.	Hide your Parkinson?	0	1	2
29.	Feel embarrassed by Parkinson?	0	1	2
30.	Worry about other people's reactions to you?	0	1	2

Thinking and Communicating

How often in the past week did you:

31.	Unexpectedly fall asleep during the day?	0	1	2
32.	Have difficulty concentrating?	0	1	2

33.	Have difficulty remembering?	0	1	2
34.	Feel people were harming you?	0	1	2
35.	Have bad dreams or hallucinations?	0	1	2
36.	Have difficulty speaking?	0	1	2
37.	Have difficulty reading?	0	1	2
38.	Feel ignored?	0	1	2

Social Support

How often in the past week did you:

39.	Have difficulty with personal relationships?	0	1	2
40.	Lack support from your spouse or partner?	0	1	2
41.	Lack support from family or friends?	0	1	2
42.	Worry about drug or medical bills?	0	1	2

Body Functions

How often in the past week did you:

43.	Have difficulty having sex?	0	1	2
44.	Have difficulty urinating?	0	1	2
45.	Have constipation?	0	1	2
46.	Drool?	0	1	2
47.	Feel dizzy or light-headed?	0	1	2
48.	Feel short of breath?	0	1	2
49.	Feel too hot or too cold?	0	1	2
50.	Have painful muscle aches or spasms?	0	1	2

Calculate Your Mobility Index: This is the sum of your score on the Mobility and Activities of Daily Living sections. ___________

Calculate Your Emotional Index: This is the sum of your score on the Emotional State, Thinking and Communicating, and Social Support sections. ___________

Calculate Your Autonomic Index (for the autonomic nervous system): This is the score on the Body Functions section. ___________

Get Your Quality of Life Score: This is the sum of your score on the Mobility Index, Emotional Index, and Autonomic Index sections. ___________

Independent of your score on the Quality of Life Scale, how do you rate your quality of life: good or bad? If it's bad, examine the relationship of your Mobility Index to your Emotional Index and your Autonomic Index and see where you can improve.

The following case report illustrates the difficulty in diagnosing PD. This report and subsequent reports are based on real people — but each report is a composite of several people. You'll recognize Anna but won't be able to speak to her.

Anna, a 57-Year-Old Woman Recently Diagnosed with Parkinson

I was 57 years old when I noticed the tremor. It affected my right hand — it wasn't there all the time, only when I was upset. I didn't think much of it — my grandmother had a tremor and she lived to 90 — and lived alone! Only later did I realize she had Benign Essential Tremor and Benign Essential Tremor isn't Parkinson. I'm a librarian, I read a lot and I know about Parkinson disease: the Pope has it, Muhammad Ali has it; goodness, Adolf Hitler had it. But I couldn't have it — could I?

Bruce, my husband, is an insurance agent. We always planned carefully. We put our two children through college — without going into debt. We exercised, we didn't smoke, we ate nourishing meals. We planned to retire when I was 60 and travel: China, Japan, Korea — Mongolia. So I couldn't have Parkinson. It sounds foolish — but Parkinson wasn't in our plans.

The tremor didn't bother me. I didn't hide it but Bruce and I didn't discuss it. We share but we don't invade each other's privacy. Then my daughter Kathy, a nurse, noticed the tremor and insisted I see a doctor: a neurologist. "Perhaps," she said, "the tremor is Parkinson."

I was anxious and scared and I insisted Bruce and Kathy come with me because if I had Parkinson I wanted my family nearby. The neurologist was young — and well trained. He had me fill out many forms and spent a long time asking me questions, some of them silly I thought. Like, "Do you have difficulty turning in bed?"

"What," I said, "does difficulty turning in bed have to do with Parkinson?"

"In Parkinson," he explained, "the limbs aren't paralyzed, they're lazy — they can but don't want to move. When you're lying in bed, looking at the ceiling, and you turn toward your left side automatically without realizing it, you swing your right arm and use it to "flip" yourself over. If you don't swing your right arm — and you don't — you may have difficulty turning in bed."

He diagnosed Parkinson on the basis of my tremor and my not swinging my right arm when I walked or when I turned in bed. He said Parkinson begins silently — 2 to 5 years before it's diagnosed. Later when we went home and watched the movies from Kathy's wedding two years ago — I wasn't swinging my right arm.

The neurologist asked us about taking part in a trial of a drug called Deprenyl. We hadn't heard about the trial — it was before the Internet. He explained that the drugs for Parkinson help the symptoms, but that Deprenyl might halt the progression of Parkinson. When we finally decided to take part — we couldn't because the trial was over-subscribed. In retrospect it didn't matter because although Deprenyl's a useful drug it doesn't halt Parkinson's progression.

I decided not to take any drug. I read more, called the National Parkinson Foundation (1-800-327-4545) and received many helpful booklets — and periodic updates. Bruce and I joined a support group. Although Bruce and I learned a lot I insisted we leave. There were too many "old" people, too many people with advanced disease. I wasn't "old" and my disease wasn't advanced. I should've been more willing to give and share — but I was scared. I hadn't been scared before I was diagnosed — but once I became a person with Parkinson, it was different. I found comfort in my husband, my family, my doctor, and in learning everything I could. I'm not religious but I began to read the Bible. It's a resource — and a balm. It fortified me in my quest to understand. From Ecclesiastes:

THE HEART OF THE WISE IS IN THE HOUSE OF MOURNING,
BUT THE HEART OF THE FOOLS IS IN THE HOUSE OF MIRTH.
IT IS BETTER TO HEAR THE REBUKE OF THE WISE,
THAN TO HEAR THE SONG OF FOOLS.
DO NOT BE QUICK TO ANGER, FOR ANGER LODGES IN THE BOSOM OF FOOLS.

Do not say, "Why were the former days better than
these?"
For it is not from wisdom that you ask this.
Wisdom is as good as an inheritance,
And gives life to the one who possesses it.

My Mobility Index is 11 (out of 40 points).
My Emotional Index is 9 (out of 44 points).
My Autonomic Index is 2 (out of 16 points).
My total score on the Quality of Life Scale is 22%.
I consider my Quality of Life as good.

Coming to Terms with the Diagnosis

If you've been diagnosed with PD you may feel many conflicting emotions. You may fear becoming physically, emotionally, and economically dependent on others. Or you may worry because money you've saved for retirement may have to go toward paying medical expenses. You may think you no longer control your future, or that you're alone, isolated. All of these concerns are normal, however, there are things you can and should do to take control over PD.

Your First Reaction — Denial

Your first reaction to being diagnosed with PD may be no reaction. You may wonder if you heard it right or if the diagnosis is correct. Such a reaction gives you time to digest the news and formulate a response. Or your first reaction may be relief — you know there's something wrong. It's not a brain tumor or a stroke, and it's not your imagination. Or you may deny the diagnosis.

"Nobody in my family has it," you say, "I'm sure it's stress. If I re-arrange my schedule, exercise regularly, pay attention to what I eat, and get a good night's sleep, my symptoms will go away."

Although exercise, nutrition, stress management, and rest are important, they won't cure PD.

Your Second Reaction — Fear and Anxiety

Realizing you have PD can make you fearful and anxious. You and your family have no idea what to expect — so you think the worst. You may fear losing your job, losing your friends, and most of all, losing your independence. These are honest reasons for being fearful or anxious. But there is an excellent way to master fear: learn as much as you can about PD. Talk with people who have PD and have gone through what you're going through. They can tell you what worked — or didn't. Find resources, information, workshops, and support groups that can help you understand PD. As an example, the National Parkinson Foundation has more than 1,000 support groups throughout the United States and a Web page (www.parkinson.org) where you can ask questions about PD.

If fear and anxiety aren't recognized they'll show up as hostility and resentment. You'll wonder what sin you committed to deserve PD. You'll become angry and direct your anger at people you love. You'll snap at minor slights or disappointments. If this happens, stop, think, and do the following:

- Recognize that having PD does not excuse being angry at others. Facing the reasons for behavior is the beginning of self-awareness. And self-awareness is the first step in coping with, adjusting to, and eventually controlling PD.
- Understand that loved ones are also upset because you have PD, and are trying to be supportive. Realize they may not know how to be helpful or supportive. Don't be afraid to tell them. Don't be afraid to talk. Everyone will benefit.
- Learn healthy ways to channel anger. Talk honestly and frankly with your spouse, a friend, or a counselor. Start by connecting with the people around you. For example, if you hesitate or "freeze" while walking, people may be puzzled. Rather than being angry, hostile, or resentful when they stare, say, "I have PD, and occasionally, I get stuck and can't move; it'll pass in a few minutes."

Your Third Reaction — Depression

Anger and resentment, especially if unrecognized, are often followed by sadness, despair, and helplessness. These are symptoms of depression — which is common in PD. If you find yourself crying frequently, withdrawing from day-to-day activities, or sleeping too much or too little, you may be depressed. Seek help — there are treatments.

A risk in accepting help for the physical aspects of your PD is that you'll become dependent on others. To lessen this retain as much responsibility for yourself as you can. By doing as much as you can for yourself, you'll feel better about yourself. The following story illustrates the difficulties in coming to terms with PD.

Melvin, 62-year-old State Senator Diagnosed with Parkinson

I was 62 years old when I "came out of the closet" and announced I had Parkinson. I'm a state senator and everyone knows me: I make things happen, I get things done. And I could be governor. So when I was diagnosed five years ago and I told my staff they said, "Don't say anything, you'll never get re-elected."

"Why?" I asked. "FDR had polio and he was President."

"Polio," they said, "isn't a brain disease. Parkinson is. Polio doesn't get worse. Parkinson does. People will see you shake and they'll think you're drunk — or senile."

I knew they were wrong. Believe it or not — I tell the truth. My wife agreed. But my staff was adamant. "They're more afraid of losing their jobs," my wife said, "than you are of losing yours."

But it wasn't just about me or my staff. A lot of people and programs depended on me. So I said nothing. And the drugs kept my symptoms under control — and hidden. I wasn't lying — just not talking."

The disease had started with stiffness and pain in my left shoulder. I played football in college and had injured my left shoulder. So when it became stiff and hurt, I was certain it was arthritis. My doctor agreed. He prescribed anti-inflammatory drugs, physical therapy, massage, acupuncture. But the stiffness and pain continued. Soon I had trouble using the arm: it was stiff and slow moving. So my doctor sent me to an orthopedist. She examined me: strength, reflexes, sensation — all normal. She obtained an MRI — also normal. Then she injected me with cortisone. When that failed she referred me to a neurologist. But when she saw the fright in my eyes, she reassured me and said, "It's probably a pinched nerve."

I was relieved until I saw the neurologist. He was bright, quick, insightful — and insensitive. "It's not a pinched nerve," he said, "it's Parkinson."

"Parkinson?" I said. "You mean I have Janet Reno's disease? But she shakes and I don't."

"Thirty percent of people don't shake," he replied.

"Will I shake? I can't afford to shake."

"Senator," he said, "you can't pass a law to stop shaking. It's not in your power."

"I want a second opinion," I replied.

"Absolutely," he said, "But don't just see anyone. Here are the names of the best."

Two second opinions later and I knew I had Parkinson disease. I returned to the first neurologist. I hadn't liked his manner, but he was direct and honest. And as I later realized it wasn't his manner, it was his diagnosis I didn't like. He knew what he was talking about. He pointed out I had trouble walking. My wife had noticed it: unsteadiness, an occasional shuffle. Because I was unsteady, and at risk of falling, he started me on Sinemet. My wife and I had read a lot and we thought you didn't start with Sinemet. But he insisted. "It's the best drug," he said, "the most rapidly acting, and it'll stop you from falling."

For four years I took controlled-release Sinemet CR (long-acting Sinemet) three times a day and it was a miracle, the stiffness and pain in my left shoulder disappeared, I no longer shuffled, no one — I thought — knew I had Parkinson. Then, I noticed each dose didn't last as long — I shuffled before the next dose. "I could give you more Sinemet," the neurologist said, "and you'll do well for a while. But it's better to combine Sinemet with a COMT inhibitor, Comtan. Comtan blocks an enzyme, COMT, that breaks down Sinemet — doubling Sinemet's effectiveness. You take Comtan with each dose of Sinemet."

It worked, I felt as well as I had a year ago. Then I was asked to run for governor. I couldn't do that — not without telling people. So my wife and I called a press conference and we announced I had Parkinson. I was relieved — and so were my constituents. One reporter said, "Parkinson — is that all? We'd seen you stagger and thought you were drunk."

We — my wife and I — decided I shouldn't run for governor. So she ran and was elected. My wife and I are religious people. I took the Quality of Life after I decided not to run for governor.

My Mobility Index is 15 (out of 40 points).

My Emotional Index is 2 (out of 44 points).

My Autonomic Index is 3 (out of 16 points).

My total score on the Quality of Life Scale is 20%.

I consider my Quality of Life as good.

My wife and I read the Bible daily. It's a been comfort to us. I like to quote from Ecclesiasticus:

> IF YOU WANT TO SERVE GOD, PREPARE YOURSELF FOR AN ORDEAL.
> BE SINCERE OF HEART, AND DO NOT BE ALARMED WHEN DANGER COMES.
> BELIEVE IN GOD, DO NOT LEAVE GOD, WHATEVER HAPPENS, ACCEPT IT.
> REMEMBER, GOLD IS TESTED IN THE FIRE, AND THE STEADFAST IN THE FURNACE.
> TRUST GOD AND GOD WILL UPHOLD YOU.
> DO NOT ABANDON YOURSELF TO SORROW, DO NOT TORMENT YOURSELF WITH ANGER.
> JOY IS WHAT GIVES LENGTH OF DAYS WHILE ANGER SHORTENS THEM.

Franklin D. Roosevelt is a prime example of a person who triumphed over the physical limitations of an illness. In 1922, when he was 40 years old, in the prime of life, at the peak of his career, after he'd been nominated for and run for vice president — he was crippled by polio. Confined to a wheelchair, unable to walk except with long, heavy leg braces and crutches, he fought his physical limitations. In 1928, he ran for and was elected governor of New York and in 1932, he was elected president. In the next 12 years, while confined to a wheelchair, he brought America out of the Great Depression and led it to triumph in history's ugliest and most dangerous war. Always remember his advice: "There is nothing to fear but fear itself!"

Should I Tell the People I Work with I've Been Diagnosed with PD?

Although it's illegal, some employers find ways to release workers with PD. If this is a concern you should speak with a lawyer knowledgeable about the Americans with Disabilities Act before discussing your PD with your employer or anyone at work. Consider the following story from Anna. "I was working as a librarian. My symptoms were mild and I didn't have to move around so I didn't feel the need to tell anyone. But as my symptoms increased I knew I couldn't keep hiding them. At first I was afraid to tell my boss because I didn't know if he'd fire me. But I told him and was surprised when he offered me a part-time job, which was easier and more pleasant."

Many people, like Anna, work for years after they're diagnosed. Others are able to work after making a few adjustments. If your symptoms are noticeable, you may want to tell your employer because it may open lines of communication. The symptoms you think are secret — usually aren't. When you decide to tell people you have PD — it will help them understand what you're going through. Remember, people who care about you and want to help have to know how they can help.

People with PD — the "pros" — offer these suggestions for newcomers to PD:

- *Tackle one problem at a time.*
- *Recognize that living with PD is difficult — not impossible.*
- *Learn, Learn, Learn!*
- *Accept PD — and live your life to the fullest.*
- *Network, Network, Network!*
- *Be positive.*
- *Let others help, but stay independent.*
- *Plan, Plan, Plan.*
- *Relationships change — but you're still you.*
- *Reduce stress, Reduce stress, Reduce stress.*
- *Believe in yourself, read the Bible, and believe in God.*

The Primary Symptoms of Parkinson Disease

There are four primary or main symptoms of PD. To diagnose PD you must have at least two primary symptoms. Secondary symptoms, discussed in Chapter 2, are combinations of primary symptoms or uncommon or minor symptoms.

1. Tremor

Tremor is the most characteristic symptom of PD and is the first symptom in 75% of people with PD. It appears as a "beating" or oscillating movement, usually of the hands, occasionally of the feet or chin. The movement is regular, 4 to 6 beats per second, and is rhythmic, each movement resembles the other. The tremor usually appears when the muscles of the hands or feet are relaxed, when they're not moving, when they're at rest. Hence the name: *resting tremor.* The tremor usually, but not always, decreases or disappears when the muscles of the hands or feet contract during movement. The resting tremor of PD typically begins on one side of the body, for example the left hand, and, later, spreads to the other side of the body. The tremor usually looks like someone is rolling a cigar, or coin, or a pill between his thumb and index finger. Hence the name "pill-rolling" tremor. The tremor is usually worse during periods of emotional or physical stress. In 20% of people with PD, the tremor is also present, or only present, during movement. This is like the tremor in another condition often confused with PD: Benign Essential Tremor, discussed in Chapter 5. Tremor, because it's driven, in part, by anxiety, may not respond as fully to drugs for Parkinson disease. Anti-cholinergic drugs (Artane, Akineton, Cogentin), Sinemet plus Comtan, and dopamine agonists (Mirapex, Permax, Requip) are helpful.

2. Rigidity

The rigidity of PD is described as stiffness or hardness of the muscles. Normally muscles contract, harden, as they move and relax, soften, as they rest. In rigidity the muscles of an affected limb stay hard as if they have contracted — when they have not. Stretching the limb is difficult. People with rigidity do not swing their arms while walking. The mask-like or expressionless face so characteristic of PD results, in part, from rigidity of the facial muscles.

Rigidity may be confused with *spasticity.* In spasticity, like rigidity, the muscles act as though they have contracted when they haven't. The hardness of spasticity has a quality that's different from rigidity. Spasticity is caused by strokes or injuries to specific brain regions, regions different from those causing rigidity. Spasticity is not a symptom of Parkinson. Rigidity may be confused with *dystonia.* In dystonia the muscles are hard or twisted because they're contracted. Dystonia can occur with or without Parkinson, but may be the first symptom of Parkinson — especially in teenagers. Dystonia, in Parkinson, may also be related to too much or too little medication. Dystonia can be painful: as painful as a pulled muscle or a charley horse.

Your doctor will test you for rigidity. First you'll be asked to relax your arms and legs. Then, your doctor will flex and extend your arms and legs. If your doctor feels resistance while moving your arm or leg, rigidity is present. Many people with PD have "cogwheel rigidity," in which the arm or leg "catches" during movement, resembling the way a cog catches in a wheel. "Cogwheel" rigidity results from a tremor superimposed on a contracting muscle. The small illegible handwriting and the decreased eye-blinking of people with Parkinson are related to rigidity. Sinemet plus Comtan, and dopamine agonists (Mirapex, Permax, Requip) are helpful.

3. Bradykinesia

Bradykinesia means slow (brady) movement (kinesia). Associated with the slowness is an incompleteness of movement, a difficulty in initiating movement, and an arrest of on-going movement. Bradykinesia is the most prominent and, usually, the most disabling symptom of Parkinson. People with bradykinesia have difficulty walking and changing positions. The slowness and incompleteness of movement associated with bradykinesia can also affect speech and swallowing. Sinemet plus Comtan and dopamine agonists are helpful.

4. Postural Instability

Postural instability is described as a lack of balance or unsteadiness while standing or changing positions. Often, care partners notice these changes before the person with Parkinson. People who are affected may have difficulty getting out of bed or keeping their balance while turning suddenly. Some of the things they did automatically, such as righting, or correcting themselves after being bumped or pushed, or after they trip, are difficult — and they may fall. Many of these corrective movements are controlled by postural reflexes. These are located deep in the brain and may be affected in PD. Postural instability does not usually respond to medication. Postural instability makes you more vulnerable to tripping or falling. However, you can compensate, in part, for your lack of balance by learning new ways to move and support yourself. Physical and occupational therapists can help.

The Anatomy and Chemistry of Parkinson Disease

The Substantia Nigra

In 1919, 102 years after Parkinson described the disease, Tretiakoff found a loss of pigmented nerve cells in *the midbrain:* a region midway between the spinal cord (the effector of movement) and the cortex (the thinking part of the brain). The loss of pigmented cells is in the *substantia nigra* (literally *the black, nigra, substance*) (See Figure 1.1). There are 400,000 nerve cells in the nigra and they begin pigmenting after birth and are fully pigmented at age 18 years. The pigment in the nigra differs from the pigment in our skins. Albinos, Caucasians, and African Americans have equal amounts of pigment in their nigra.

In 1913 Lewy described a pink-staining round body, the Lewy body, within the cell body of dying nerve cells (Figure 1.2). Although Lewy bodies are found in people unaffected by PD and in a few, rare diseases other than PD, the Lewy body is considered essential for diagnosing PD. The Lewy body contains at least three proteins: *alpha-synnuclein, parkin,* and *ubiquitin.* The functions of these proteins are just becoming known.

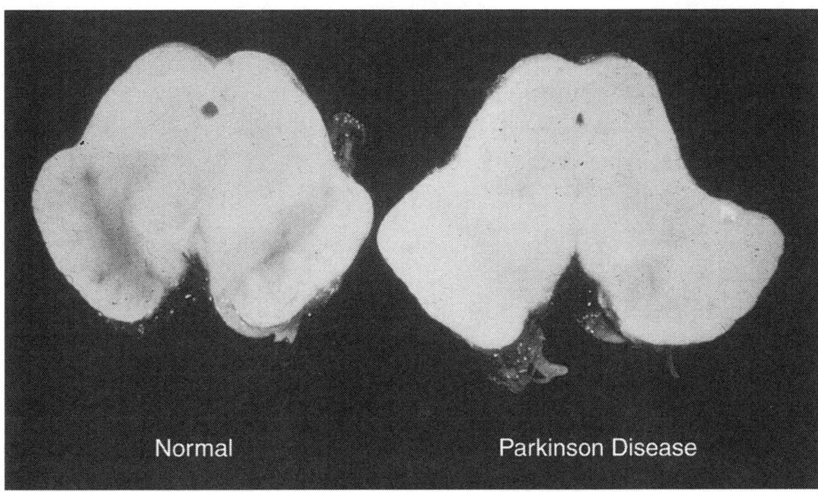

Figure 1.1 The Substantia Nigra, Part of the Brain, in Normal and PD

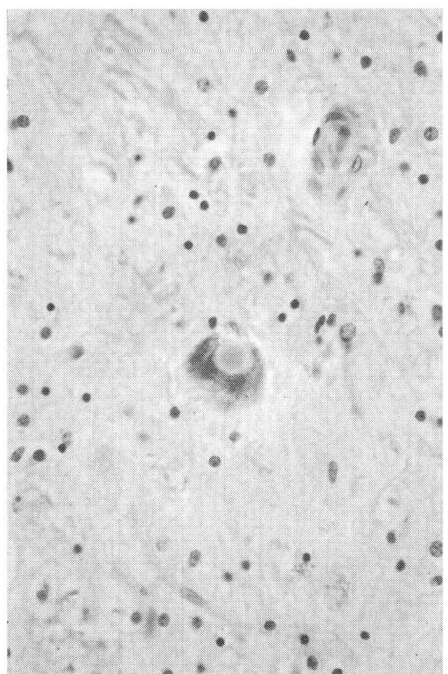

Figure 1.2 Lewy Bodies in a Neuron from the Substantia Nigra in PD

The symptoms of PD appear after about 240,000 cells in the nigra die: 60% of the total. In normal, unaffected people perhaps 2,400 cells in the nigra die yearly. If you live 100 years and lose 240,000 cells you're at risk for PD. In PD the loss of cells in the nigra accelerates — more than 2,400 cells die each year — how many more is unknown. It's also unknown why the loss accelerates.

The loss of nerve cells in a small region, the nigra, results in a loss of dopamine in a larger region, the striatum, which in turn disrupts a larger, interconnected brain network: the basal ganglia.

The Interconnections of the Brain: The Basal Ganglia

Paralleling the loss of cells in the nigra is a loss of the chemical dopamine in another region of the brain called the striatum (Figure 1.3). The loss of dopamine in the striatum was discovered by Oleh Hornykiewicz and Walter Birkmayr in 1960. The cells from the nigra reach upward to the striatum through the nigro-striatal pathway, a pathway discovered by Anka Dahlstrom and Kjell Fuxe in 1972. In the striatum the fibers from the nigra mingle with fibers that reach downward from the cortex. This co-mingling of fibers gives a stripped appearance to the striatum hence its name from the Latin *the stripped substance.*

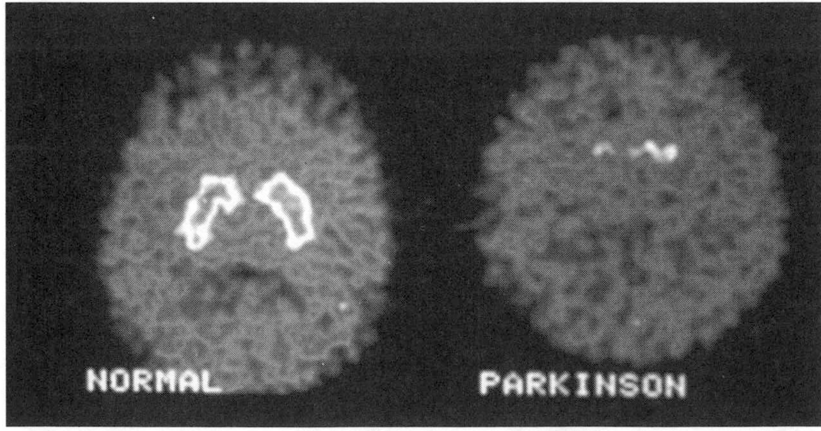

Figure 1.3 *Positron Emission Tomography Showing Reduced Dopamine*

The fibers from the nigra contact specialized proteins, the dopamine receptors, that are located on the bodies of the cells of the striatum. There are at least five types of dopamine receptors. In the striatum there are two types of dopamine receptors called the D-1 and D-2, each specific for a different type of cell in the striatum. The fibers from the cortex contact specialized proteins, called glutamate receptors that are on the bodies of the cells of the striatum, the cells that contain the D-1 and D-2 receptors. Understanding the relationship of the D-1 to the D-2 receptors and both of them to the glutamate receptors will enable us to devise new and more effective treatments for PD.

Fibers from D-1 containing cells reach down through the *direct pathway* to a pale, globe-like region of the brain called the *globus pallidus* from the Latin pale globe. These fibers contact nerve cells whose fibers, in turn, reach another region of the brain called *the thalamus* from the Latin for chamber or room. Fibers from D-2 containing cells reach down through the indirect pathway first to the subthalamus, then the pallidum then the thalamus. Fibers from nerve cells in the thalamus then reach up to the cortex. Understanding the relationship of these pathways has resulted in operations, pallidotomy, thalamotomy, and deep-brain stimulation that are changing the treatment of PD. Most investigators believe the primary event causing PD is the loss of nigral cells. This results in overactivity of subthalamic and pallidal nerve cells — an overactivity akin to excessive braking of an automobile — resulting in slowed movements. A few investigators believe the primary event is overactivity of the subthalamic and pallidal nerve cells.

CHAPTER
2

Parkinson: A Disease of Moving — Again

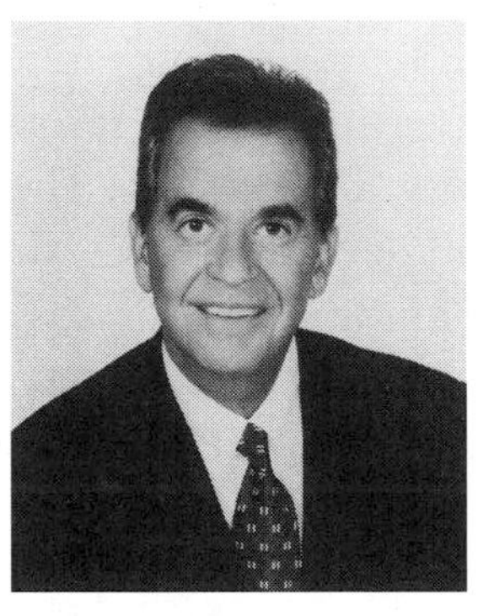

Dick Clark,
Television personality, Producer

"My father had Parkinson. He lived to be one month shy of 93. It was with him for twenty some-odd years. The first time we became aware of it was when my mother noticed it. I guess that's usual — the partner is the first to notice it. My father was an athlete. He was quite a handsome man. He lived a full life, and was very smart. As the Parkinson progressed, he didn't lose a great deal. He lost a little bit of his physical mobility, but his mind remained remarkably intact. He was wonderful. He remained the patriarch of the family. Everybody turned to him for advice. Nobody looked at him as a victim or as a patient, or felt sorry for him. We adapted our lifestyle a little bit to help him. So it's not the end of the world. The point is you never lose your function. You never lose the respect of the people around you.

"We made adaptations to make my dad's life easier. Although he lived alone for a number of years after my mom passed away, we finally convinced him to move in with us. We had a large house, and as a matter of fact, we built that house with his Parkinson in mind. I said to the builder (because my dad was having a little difficulty walking at that point) 'Put a double railing on the stairs so that he can hold on to both sides.' That worked. For the bathroom, I told the builder, 'Build a shower so small that he can't fall down, and put railings around.' It was a little inconvenient for the average person but he could get in and out easily.

"When his finger movement became difficult, I said, 'Pappy, don't worry about that, I'll make you some shirts with buttons on the front, but they'll have Velcro on the back.' There are a lot of things that you can do that are disguised adaptations of normal clothing and only you and the patient know they are making life a little bit easier.

"I think what you have to do early on as a family member is adjust to the fact that the person is eventually going to change. You may have a little difficulty understanding the speech pattern. Maybe he or she won't speak loudly enough and you're always saying, 'What, what, what?' Or they take these little tiny baby steps, and you say, 'Come on, just move those legs and . . . .' As a person in or around it, you have to be a little more patient and a little more understanding. You've got to say, 'We don't care about that stuff. It's having you around, and with us, sharing your advice and whatever you can contribute to the family — that's important to us.'

"I think with any problem we face, whether it's physical or mental, if you can find other people who share the problem and swap stories, swap solutions, it's always helpful — you know you're not alone. It can strike young, it can strike old, it can strike white, it can strike black, rich or poor — it's totally indiscriminate, but you're not alone.

"As I read this book, I said to my wife, 'Wouldn't this have been handy if we'd only known what we were doing?' We did everything ad lib."

The Secondary Symptoms of Parkinson That Affect Mobility

Secondary symptoms that affect mobility are called "secondary" because they arise from a combination of two or more primary symptoms, or are less common or less disabling than primary symptoms. Among the secondary symptoms that affect mobility are difficulty walking, freezing or hesitation when walking, difficulty turning, stooped posture, difficulty speaking, and difficulty writing.

Walking

Difficulty walking arises from a combination of rigidity, slowness of movement, and postural instability. The rigidity and slowness of movement affect the muscles of the foot, calf, thigh, hip, and one or both sides of the body, as well as the muscles of the pelvis and spine. In PD, difficulty walking may occur early or late in the illness. The difficulty consists of taking short steps, often with the heel of one foot not clearing the toe of the other. Occasionally the short steps run together causing you to run forward or, occasionally, backward. The short steps result from slowness and lack of movement of the legs and feet. The difficulty walking also consists of not swinging one or both arms. Swinging the arms helps maintain balance and helps in propelling the feet forward. The lack of arm swing results from rigidity of the arms and from loss of associated movements. Associated movements are programmed into the brain so that when you put your foot forward your arm moves as well. These movements are lost in PD. The combination of short steps and lack of arm swing make walking even harder. The short steps and lack of arm swing respond to Sinemet plus Comtan or a dopamine agonist.

Is the Difficulty Walking Caused by Something Other Than Parkinson?

People with PD who have difficulty walking and do not respond to medication should be checked for other diseases or conditions that cause difficulty walking. Among these are:

1. Arthritis of the hips and knees.
2. Diseases of the arteries in the legs.
3. Diseases of the nerves in the legs, or neuropathy, may have several causes from diabetes to vitamin B deficiency to alcohol to toxic chemicals.
4. Diseases of the spinal cord. From a slipped disc in the lower spine, to a bony spur compressing the upper spine, diseases of the upper spine are often overlooked as the cause of difficulty walking in PD people — especially when they occur without pain.
5. Diseases of the brain from multiple, small and silent strokes to excess fluid on the brain (hydrocephalus) to blood clots and brain tumors can be responsible for difficulty walking.

These diseases may be separated from PD and from each other through a careful history, a detailed physical and neurological examination, a variety of blood tests, and an MRI of the upper spine and brain.

Stooped Posture

Stooped posture, which accompanies and contributes to difficulty walking, arises from rigidity or dystonia of the muscles of the spine. In some the stoop is so great they walk with their eyes glued to the floor. The stooped posture results from either the center-of-gravity being thrown forward, causing the person to stoop to catch-up, or from a constant, uneven and powerful pull of the muscles of the front of the spine over those of the back of the spine.

The stooping itself may result in difficulty walking. The spine is a fulcrum around which the hip, thigh, and buttock muscles generate the power needed for walking. If the spine bends or stoops forward, the hip, thigh, and buttock muscles lose power. To show this:

1. Stand and bend at the waist, stare at the floor.
2. Walk while bending at the waist with your eyes on the floor. Less power is generated with your hip, thigh, and buttock muscles forcing you to walk with short steps. The stooping may be partly corrected by Sinemet plus Comtan or a dopamine agonist; it may also be treated with corrective exercises. The exercises consist of the following:

    - Reach your hands over your head, grab and hold onto a "chinning" bar; pull yourself up slowly without actually lifting your feet off the floor. This exercise stretches the muscles of your spine; it should be done at least 10 times, at least twice a day.
    - Stand with your arms behind your back, your right hand grabbing your left wrist; pull down. This movement forces your shoulders up and straightens your spine. This should be done 10–20 times, at least three times a day, a total of 30–60 times a day.
    - Sit on a stationary bicycle and pedal (not fast) for 30 minutes a day while fixing your eyes on a picture or TV screen above eye level. This forces your shoulders up and straightens your spine.

Freezing

Freezing is an inability to start walking, called "start hesitation," or a sudden inability to continue walking, called "stop hesitation," like a computer glitch that freezes the screen. Start hesitation may occur separate from or together with stop hesitation. These two types of freezing may involve different circuits or pathways in the brain. Start hesitation usually responds to Sinemet plus Comtan or a dopamine agonist. Stop hesitation may or may not respond to Sinemet or a dopamine agonist. The inability to continue walking usually occurs while turning or coming to a door. One theory on why people freeze is that the brain "sees" the length of each stride. People walk with a different stride on level versus hilly ground or in open versus closed spaces. When walking on level ground the brain goes into "autopilot" and depending on what it sees, one step automatically follows the next. When you reach an obstacle — a hole in the ground, another person, a doorway — you must change stride length. A person with PD may be unable to switch from autopilot to another program, and, like a faulty computer, freezes. In some people, even thinking of changing stride length when approaching a door is enough to cause freezing.

Anxiety increases freezing. People with PD who are anxious freeze more frequently. Once they freeze, anxiety increases and they are more likely to freeze again. For some, freezing is like a panic attack with sweating, a faster beating heart, and shortness of breath. Treating anxiety may decrease freezing. People who freeze learn a variety of tricks to get moving again. Most tricks involve straightening the spine. Learning a trick that breaks the freeze reduces anxiety. Some of the more common tricks include:

- Imagining a line on the floor and trying to step over it
- Humming a tune
- Counting in a marching cadence
- Stepping over a foot or object in front of you
- Rocking from side-to-side to get started
- Summoning your willpower and taking one long step forward

Freezing and Fluctuations: Some people with PD on Sinemet fluctuate, they have on-and-off periods and may freeze in one of these periods. The freezing in the off period usually responds to more Sinemet or the addition of Comtan. The freezing in the on period may or may not respond to more medication. This suggests there are different types of freezing involving different circuits and pathways.

Canes, Sticks, and Walkers: A cane or a walker that is too low forces you to bend, making you take short steps. Whatever support gained from the cane or walker is defeated by bending the spine. Try a walking stick rather than a cane. The stick should be level with your shoulder and held in a straight line from your shoulder to your hand, forcing the shoulders up and straightening out the spine. Remember Moses, who was 120 years of age, used a walking stick not a cane, and he walked from Egypt, across the Sinai, to Jordan. He couldn't have done it with a cane. Be careful, however, a walking stick isn't for everyone, some people have less balance with a walking stick. If there's a question, use both under the supervision of a physical therapist.

A walker should be high enough to prevent stooping. If there's a question as to whether your walker's right for you, go to a supermarket and walk using a shopping cart. The handles of the cart are high, forcing you to walk straight. If you're more comfortable walking with the cart than your walker, your walker isn't right for you because it may be too low or its wheels may be too small. The smaller the wheels the more energy you use to push the walker.

Speaking

Speaking may be affected in Parkinson. Congressman Morris Udall of Arizona had difficulty speaking. This was especially noticeable in Mo, a gifted public speaker. Mo made up for his difficulty speaking with his ability to use his eyes, his hand gestures, and his smile. His nonverbal communication could be as loud as thunder in the desert.

Earl Ubell, the renowned health editor of *Parade Magazine,* takes speech therapy, although his voice is unaffected, because, as he says, "I don't want my voice to become weak. Speech therapy, I'm convinced, helps it stay the same."

Difficulty speaking arises from rigidity, bradykinesia, and less often tremor of the muscles of speech production. To understand how PD can affect your speaking you must understand how speech is produced. There are four parts (Figure 2.1).

1. Breathing — the "fuel" of speaking. At rest, your lungs move air in and out of your throat, mouth, and nose. The lungs

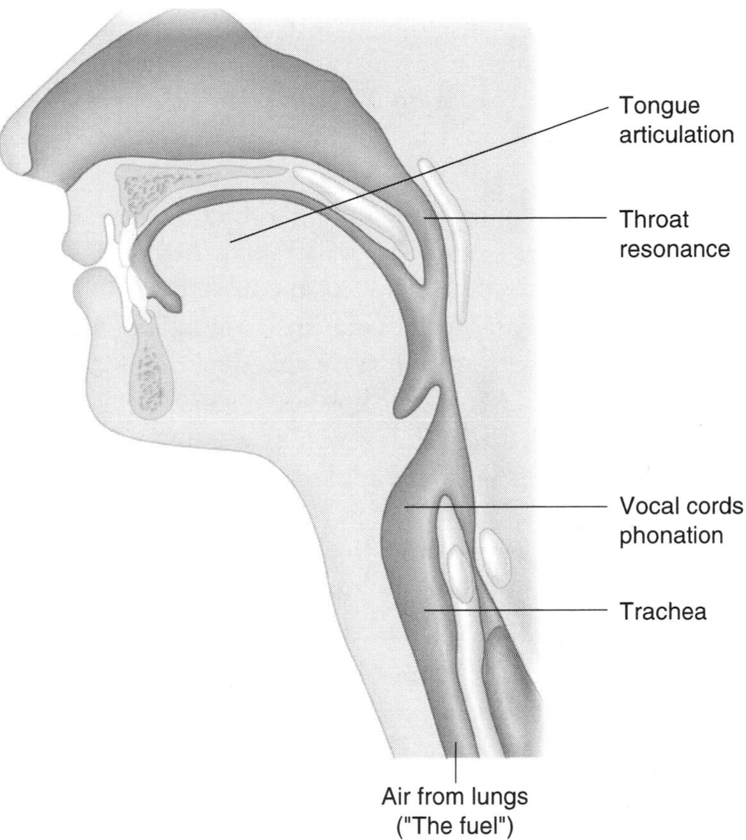

Figure 2.1 *How Speech Is Produced*

are a "bellows;" the muscles of the chest wall, belly, and the diaphragm work together to suck air into the lungs during inspiration, and force air out of the lungs during expiration. If, as may happen in PD, your chest-wall muscles become rigid, you suck less air in and force less air out. You breathe faster, which is tiring, and shallower, which is less efficient. Your voice becomes lower. Try speaking while holding your breath — and you'll appreciate the problem. Treatment consists of learning to breathe slowly and deeply, training your voice like an opera singer.

2. Phonation — translating air into sounds. Sounds, mainly vowels, are formed from air rushing out of your lungs past your larynx (the voice box). The larynx lies just above the Adam's apple. The vocal cords lie inside the larynx. The vocal cords are muscles that open and close so quickly — they vibrate. Rigidity, dystonia, or bradykinesia of the vocal cords changes how air becomes sounds.

To appreciate what your vocal cords do — imagine your lips are your cords. Pucker your lips creating a hole and whistle. Air rushes past your lips. By changing the size and shape of the hole by curving your lips you change the sound of the whistle. If the lips are rigid — you'll have difficulty whistling. If the vocal cords become rigid or bradykinetic, as they do in PD, you'll have difficulty speaking. Sinemet plus Comtan improves mobility — including vocal cord mobility; during treatment your voice will become louder.

Tremor of the vocal cords results in a quivering, or tremulous voice. Rarely, in some people with PD, the vocal cords are dystonic and during treatment your voice, instead of getting louder, gets lower. There's a disorder called spastic dysphonia, distinct from PD, in which the vocal cords become dystonic, resulting in a low and quivering voice. Spastic dysphonia can be treated successfully with injections of botulinum toxin. Distinguishing rigidity from dystonia of the cords requires looking at the cords through a laryngoscope.

3. Resonance — "amplifying sounds in the auditorium of the mouth." Once sounds are formed in the larynx, they resonate in an amphitheater — the spaces of the throat, mouth, and nose, and the passages between the nose and throat. The muscles of these structures lengthen, shorten, dilate, and constrict, to change the shape of the spaces between the lips and larynx. Because these muscles change shape as you speak, they change the richness, the resonance, the tang, and twang of your voice. If these muscles are rigid, bradykinetic, or tremulous, your voice will be affected. To appreciate these changes hold your nose and speak or put your finger in the back of your throat and speak.

4. Articulation — the "mechanics of speaking." Articulation requires the muscles of the face, lips, tongue, and jaw. While speaking, these muscles move rapidly in a coordinated manner making for clear and precise speech. Some people with PD say they can't form or pronounce words clearly; some say their words are slurred, and some say they speak as though they're drunk or had a stroke. These changes, called *dysarthria,* differ from the changes that occur with difficulty breathing, difficulty phonating, or difficulty resonating. Dysarthria is more common in some of the Parkinson-like diseases such as Shy Drager or Progressive Supranuclear Palsy. These are discussed later. Dysarthria results from rigidity and bradykinesia of the muscles of the face, the lips, the tongue, and the jaw. To appreciate these changes hold your lips, face, or tongue and speak.

Many people with PD are unaware of their difficulty speaking. If told they speak too softly, they might reply, "It's not me, it's you — get a hearing aid." Making someone aware that they have difficulty speaking by taping them and then playing the tape back can be revealing.

Hints for people with PD who have difficulty speaking:

- Always look directly at the person to whom you're speaking.
- Eliminate all background noise while speaking.
- Be calm.

Exercises for people with PD who have difficulty speaking:

- Take a deep breath and shout: "AH." Hold the "AH" as long as you can.
- Take a deep breath and loudly sing a musical scale: "La, La, La, La, La, La, La" both going up and coming down.
- Read a magazine article out loud. No one has to be listening.

Lorraine Ramig of the University of Colorado developed an effective treatment called the *Lee Silverman Voice Treatment* (LSVT).

The treatment improves your ability to speak by strengthening the muscles of your lungs, your larynx, and your throat through speaking loudly or shouting.

Difficulty swallowing may or may not accompany difficulty speaking. Although the muscles of speaking and swallowing are similar, they're controlled differently and one function does not necessarily accompany the other. Difficulty speaking may occur early in PD, while difficulty swallowing usually occurs late in PD. Difficulty swallowing is discussed in Chapter 4.

Writing

A common symptom of PD is a change in handwriting, especially when the right hand is affected: 90% of people are right-handed and almost all write with their right hand. The difficulty writing, called *micro-graphia* (small handwriting), results from the effects of rigidity, bradykinesia, and tremor on the muscles of the arm. Difficulty writing and speaking is illustrated in the next case report.

Jack, a 60-Year-Old Lawyer with Six Years of Parkinson: Trouble Speaking and Writing

My dad, Jack Senior, had Parkinson disease — and it made a bad impression on me. When he was diagnosed Sinemet had just come out. He was treated with it and did well for a while. Then he developed dyskinesias: gyrating, twisting, turning movements of his head, chest, arms, and legs. Now we know he was overdosed — we didn't then. If there was a disease I didn't want, it was Parkinson.

My dad was in military intelligence during World War II, he met all the important people: Churchill, de Gaulle, General Marshal, Patton, Roosevelt, and Stalin — and collected their autographs. He got to question all the Nazi big shots: Göring, Hess, Field Marshal Keitel, Ribbentrop, and Speer — and collected their autographs. I became a history buff and, when I wasn't working as a lawyer, I continued his collection. Hitler, in a freakish and perverted way, fascinated me — and I collected his autographs. Examining Hitler's signature, I saw it had changed between 1933 and 1945 (when he committed suicide): the writing had become smaller, more cramped — like my dad's (See Figure 2.2). Hitler, I concluded, had Parkinson disease — and later this was shown to be so. How ironic Nature is — my dad, whom I loved, and Hitler, whom I hated, had the same disease.

It was 4 years ago, while doing my taxes and comparing my returns for the last 2 years that I noticed my signature had changed. It was smaller and more cramped! "Could I have Parkinson disease?" I asked.

"No," I replied trying to calm myself, "Nature's not that ironic."

I yelled for my wife and pointing to my signature I asked, "Do you see anything — strange?"

"Such as?" she asked.

"Such as my handwriting getting smaller?" I said.

"Like your dad's?" she replied.

I was waiting for her to say I was crazy. Her answer stunned me. "Your handwriting does look like your dad's — and you also speak like him — softly."

The next day I demanded to see a neurologist — a Parkinson specialist. His secretary thought I was a lunatic. "The doctor," she said, "doesn't handle emergencies."

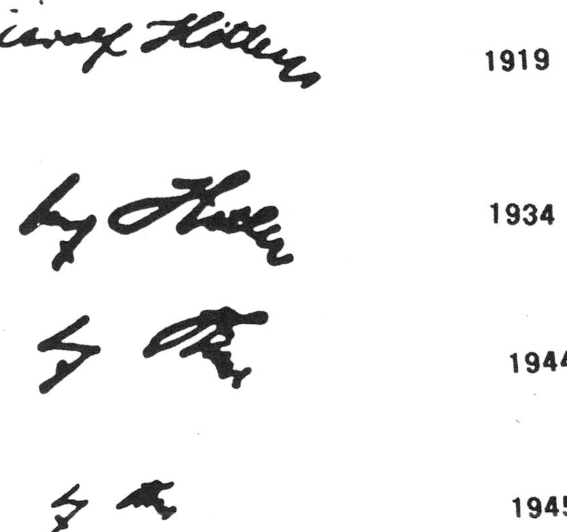

Figure 2.2 Adolf Hitler's Signature

I have a friend, Lenny, who has a Parkinson-like disease, Shy Drager, and he's a big contributor to the medical center. As a favor to Lenny, the neurologist agreed to see me the same day I called. It was after 7 P.M. when he saw me and confirmed the diagnosis. Two things bothered me. I had difficulty speaking and knew the muscles of speaking are the same as the muscles of swallowing. I wanted to know if, like my dad, I'd develop difficulty swallowing. My dad, late in his disease, had difficulty swallowing, he aspirated, developed pneumonia — and died. Was that going to happen to me?

"No," the neurologist said, "although the muscles of speech and swallowing are the same, they're controlled differently, and difficulty speaking doesn't necessarily mean difficulty swallowing."

The second question was about Sinemet. I was afraid of it. The neurologist explained that the complications of Sinemet are related to the drug's short half-life, 1.5 hours, and to the progression of the disease. "If," he said, "from the beginning you combine Sinemet with a COMT inhibitor the Sinemet lasts twice as long and some of the complications, such as dyskinesias, may not develop. In fact we're doing a study just on that."

What he said made sense, but I was still afraid. Reading my mind, he continued, "If you're afraid, we have another study in which we're using a dopamine agonist — Mirapex. Sinemet has to be changed by the brain to dopamine. The agonists don't have to be changed to anything — they mimic Sinemet. The agonists have a longer half-life but they're not as potent as Sinemet."

"Will Mirapex help my speaking?" I asked. "I'm a lawyer — I live by speaking."

"Yes," he replied.

"Will Mirapex help my handwriting?" I asked. "I go berserk whenever I sign my name — it reminds me I have Parkinson."

"Yes," he replied.

"Will Mirapex cause dyskinesias?" I asked.

"It may," he replied, "but at a later date and to a lesser degree."

"I'll sign up," I said.

"The benefits aren't forever," he said, "eventually, in 2 to 4 years, you'll need Sinemet and Comtan."

"In 2 to 4 years, I'll be ready emotionally. But not now."

Physically I've done well on Mirapex, my speaking and handwriting have improved, people don't know I have Parkinson, and I don't tell them, but emotionally I'm a mess. I'm depressed, I feel isolated, I'm anxious, I don't want to talk to my wife, and I worry about the future — about becoming like my dad. I know it's me — my attitude. I wish I had Lenny's attitude — he's physically worse than me but calm, reassured. He asked me to read the Bible and I did: the Book of Job.

PERISH THE DAY ON WHICH I WAS BORN,
AND THE NIGHT I WAS CONCEIVED.
MAY THAT DAY BE DARKNESS,
MAY NO LIGHT SHINE ON IT,
LET IT BE CURSED BY ALL,
LET DARK BE THE STARS OF ITS MORNING,
LET IT WAIT IN VAIN FOR THE LIGHT,
AND NEVER SEE THE EYES OF THE DAWN.

I recently took the Quality of Life Exam. I've a worse Quality of Life than Lenny — and physically he's worse than I.

My Mobility Index is 11 (out of 40). My mobility is under control.

My Emotional Index is 28 (out of 44). My emotions aren't under control.

My Autonomic Index is 3 (out of 16).

My total score on the Quality of Life Scale is 42%.

I consider my Quality of Life as bad.

CHAPTER

3

Parkinson: You'll Be Surprised Who Gets It

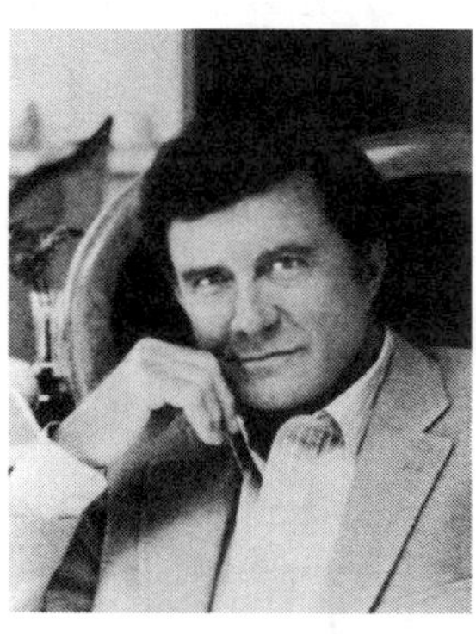

Cliff Robertson,
Actor, friend of Congressman Morris Udall

"I watched my good friend Morris Udall, Mo as we called him, suffer tremendously from Parkinson disease. He was a tall man of great stature standing at about six feet four inches. And when I'd see him in the hospital every time — and I went down regularly — he seemed to be getting smaller. The body was suffering.

"His condition became progressively worse. After a while he couldn't talk, but he could convey feelings. And I wrote a piece on my way back from seeing him one day called 'I Saw Mo Today.' Part of it reads:

'I SAW MO TODAY.

The man who loved and saved God's wilderness, who spoke for those who could not speak, who worked for those who could not work, who listened to those without counsel, who loved those without love.
I saw Mo today.
He could not stand nor speak or even smile; he just listened.
And when I squeezed his hand to go, he opened his eyes, he looked at me long, just looked, and I heard every word.'"

Parkinson in Young People

Parkinson is a disease of aging. The greatest risk factor for PD is growing old. At 70 the risk for PD is much greater than at 35. Since the perpetually young actor Michael J. Fox was diagnosed with PD before age 35, PD is no longer your grandfather's disease. Instead of children being concerned about PD in their parents, parents are concerned about PD in their children. Doctors who never considered diagnosing PD below age 35 now must.

How Common Is Parkinson in Young People?

Typical, adult-onset PD usually begins at age 60 or later. Until recently, PD starting prior to age 35 was considered rare, except in Japan. Studies in the United States and Europe report the incidence of *new* cases of people younger than 35 with PD as 10 people with PD per 1,000,000 people. As compared with the incidence of new cases of PD in all people, the occurrence of PD in people 35 or younger 200 people per 1,000,000; 20 times higher.

The prevalence of PD in people below the age of 35, the number of all people below age 35 with PD, is about 5% of all PD patients. In Japan, the prevalence of PD in people below 35 is, in some medical centers, as much as 25% of PD patients.

Is Young-Onset Parkinson Different from Adult-Onset Parkinson?

People in the United States, Europe, and Japan who develop PD between the ages of 21 and 40 are diagnosed with young-onset

PD. People who develop PD before the age of 21 are diagnosed with juvenile PD. Young-onset PD resembles, on post-mortem examination, typical adult-onset PD. Juvenile PD, however, is a mix of diseases. Half of the people with juvenile PD resemble, on post-mortem examination, typical adult-onset PD characterized by a loss of nerve cells in the substantia nigra with Lewy bodies inside the dying cells. Half of the people with juvenile PD do not resemble, on post-mortem examination, typical adult-onset PD.

The progression of symptoms in people with young-onset PD is slower than in people with typical adult-onset PD. In young-onset PD the symptoms are similar to typical adult-onset PD except, in young-onset PD dystonia, painful muscular contractions of both feet, is common. In young-onset PD, decline in intellect, difficulty thinking, and autonomic nervous system symptoms are uncommon.

Young-onset PD and juvenile PD people respond to Sinemet, and Sinemet plus Comtan, with end of Sinemet dose wearing off, and both groups may be more likely than adult-onset PD to develop wearing-off, on-off, and dyskinesias.

Jerry, a 38-Year-Old Dentist with Young-Onset Parkinson Disease

I was 35 years old when I saw the tremor in my left hand. I'm a dentist, I live by my hands — and I was scared. I was going through a painful divorce. I'd been sleeping around and my wife found out. We have three kids. When I saw the tremor I said, "It's my nerves. What else could it be at my age?"

The tremor got worse and I learned to hide it by not using my left hand while working. "It'll go away," I said. When it didn't I saw a friend of mine, a neurologist. I was stunned when he said, "You have Parkinson disease."

"Parkinson? No way," I replied, "I'm 35, Parkinson's your grandmother's disease. It's something else: anxiety or Benign Essential Tremor."

"Anxiety," he said, " doesn't affect only one side. And neither does Benign Essential Tremor."

"Then," I said, "it's a low/high calcium, or magnesium, or my thyroid."

"They don't affect only one side. And as for your age — there's Michael J. Fox."

"Jerk," I thought, "for reminding me."

"I'll check you for calcium, magnesium, and thyroid — but it's more than a tremor. Your left hand's slower than your right."

I went home, got out my neurology book, and read about Parkinson disease. It confirmed what my friend said. I asked for and got another opinion. The Parkinson specialist confirmed the diagnosis — in two minutes. For support I turned to my mother; I couldn't turn to my wife. My mother was devastated. You see, her mother had Parkinson disease — and she never told me. She was certain I'd inherited it from her or from sleeping around. She couldn't support me — emotionally, I had to support her — emotionally: she was a basket case. She kept referring to the Book of Job:

> LYING IN BED I WONDER, "WHEN WILL IT BE DAY?"
> NO SOONER UP THEN, "WHEN WILL EVENING COME?"
> AND CRAZY THOUGHTS FILL MY HEAD TILL TWILIGHT.
> SWIFTER THAN A WEAVER'S SHUTTLE MY DAYS PASS,
> AND VANISH LEAVING NO HOPE BEHIND.
> OUR LIFE IS BUT A BREATH OF AIR, AND OUR EYES WILL NEVER AGAIN SEE JOY.

I decided to help myself. But first I had to be certain, despite the opinion of two neurologists, that I had Parkinson disease. So I traveled to another city to have a PET-scan. It confirmed the diagnosis. Then I thought, "There must be a reason for my Parkinson — one that can be treated and reversed. I looked into everything. Now I know it was part of my denial — a kind of magical thinking: a quick fix. I had myself checked for "silent" strokes, a brain tumor, and venereal disease: syphilis and AIDS — because I'd been sleeping around. Blood tests and an MRI were normal. I even had a spinal tap. It was normal. Next I was certain it was the drugs I'd used in college: diet pills and marijuana. I was not reassured by the specialist: none of the drugs I'd used caused Parkinson — as far as he knew. I vowed never to use a drug unless it was medically necessary.

Then I read the reports on mercury poisoning. Mercury can cause a tremor and difficulty walking that is "distinctly different" from Parkinson. But I didn't know what "distinctly different from Parkinson" meant. So I asked the specialist.

"Distinctly different to an expert," he said, condescendingly.

"Jerk," I thought. "This won't be the first time the experts are wrong."

By now I was convinced it was mercury poisoning. I'm a dentist, I work with mercury amalgams, I have amalgams in my teeth. Perhaps the amalgams had leaked mercury into my blood and from there it had gotten into my brain. I had my blood, urine, and hair tested for mercury. Mercury poisoning is accumulative, levels in the blood and urine aren't as important as levels in the hair: meaning that mercury has accumulated there — and presumably in the brain. Since testing for mercury isn't routine I sent specimens to two different labs. Everything was normal. Nevertheless I had a friend pull all of my teeth with amalgams. Then I waited for the tremor to go away — it got worse!

My receptionist and my hygienist saw it, and I'm certain my patients, and lady friends saw it — the ones who didn't come back. I didn't know where to turn. Through the National Parkinson Foundation I found a support group in another city. I listened to a lady, Anna, tell about her "coming out" with Parkinson and how helpful her family and doctor had been. I went home and called my wife, apologized, told her about my Parkinson and she took me back! Next, I saw the dean of the dental school, and asked him for a part-time job as an instructor. Then I told my office staff, hired an associate, and told my patients. Some left but most stayed: they appreciated my honesty, they valued my judgment, and knew that if I lacked the dexterity to do something my associate would do it.

I called Anna from the support group, and got the name of her specialist and went with my wife to see him. He spent a lot of time talking to us — the other specialist hadn't. Or, to be kind, maybe I hadn't been ready to listen. Anna's doctor told us about several drugs he was testing in recently diagnosed people with Parkinson: Sinemet plus Comtan and three separate dopamine agonists: Mirapex, Permax, and Requip. And two drugs that might slow the progression of Parkinson. My wife and I haven't decided whether I should take part in a trial or whether I should be on any drug at this time. Getting our life and myself together is, at this time, a greater priority than controlling a tremor.

Recently I took the Quality of Life Examination. Six months ago, when the tremor was less, but before I started to get my life together, my Quality of Life was worse.

My Mobility Index is 4 (out of 40 points).

My Emotional Index is 17 (out of 44 points).

My Autonomic Index is 3 (out of 16 points).

My total score on the Quality of Life Scale is 24%.

I consider my Quality of Life as good — and improving.

Famous People with Parkinson — Why So Many?

The following famous people were diagnosed with PD (in alphabetical order):

Muhammad Ali
Jack Anderson, the newspaper columnist
Jim Backus, the voice of "Mr. Magoo"
Chester Bowles, former Ambassador to India
Ernie Bushmiller, creator of "Nancy" and "Sluggo"
Salvador Dali
Michael J. Fox
Francisco Franco, former leader of Spain
Adolf Hitler
Arthur Koestler, the author of "A Darkness of Noon"
Rhode Island Senator Claiborne Pell
Pope John Paul II
Sir Michael Redgrave, actor
Janet Reno, former United States Attorney General
Terry Thomas, actor
Earl Ubell, editor
Rhode Island Congressman Morris Udall
Deng Xiaoping, successor to Mao Zedong

Famous people get PD; infamous people get PD, and ordinary people get PD. But do a higher percent of famous people get PD?

Is there something about PD that leads to fame first and then PD? There are 3,500 Americans with PD per 1,000,000 people, or 0.3% of the population. What's the percent among famous people?

What Is Fame?

First ask what is fame? How is it measured? One way of measuring fame is to look at people who are selected to be on the cover of *Time* magazine. The man or woman chosen is the person, who in the opinion of *Time*'s editors is, for a week, the most newsworthy, and by implication, the most famous. It's not a measure with which everyone agrees, including the editors of the *Economist, Newsweek, Reader's Digest* or *U.S. News & World Report.* And it's a fleeting measure, there are 52 issues of *Time* each year; 52 famous men and women each year, 3,796 men and women in the 73 years since 1927, when *Time* began.

A more enduring measure of fame is being on the cover of *Time* magazine as its "Person of the Year." Choosing the person of the year as the measure of fame involves relying on the professionalism, the objectivity, and the knowledge of a particular group of editors. Ordinarily such choices, which aren't random, aren't compatible with the rules of statistical probability. There are other more objective measures of fame, such as the Nobel Prize or sainthood in the Catholic Church, but *Time* it is — and probability will sort itself out.

Between 1927 and 2000, 60 individuals appeared as *Time* Person of the Year. If people who appeared more than once are counted as one, then 48 people appeared as *Time* Person of the Year in that period. Three of the 48 have PD. The three are: Adolf Hitler, Deng Xiaoping, and Pope John Paul II. Three out of 48 is 6.2% or 20 times the prevalence of PD in the United States.

Among the 60 people who appeared as *Time* Person of the Year, are 11 who appeared more than once. The 11 are:

Winston Churchill
Deng Xiaoping
Dwight D. Eisenhower

Mikhail Gorbachev
Lyndon B. Johnson
George C. Marsha
Richard M. Nixon
Ronald Reagan
Franklin D. Roosevelt
Josef Stalin
Harry S Truman

One of the 11, Deng Xiaoping, has PD. One out of 11 is 9.0% or 22 times the prevalence of PD in the United States.

What Is There About Parkinson and Fame?

Do famous people, like ordinary people, get PD because it's a disease of maturity? A disease that allows its victims sufficient time to become famous — then suffer? It's not a disease of birth, infancy, or childhood; a disease that doesn't allow its victims time to become famous. It's not Down Syndrome or childhood AIDS. PD is not a disease that destroys the developing or maturing brain. The peak onset is at age 60 years. And, by age 60 years, famous people, and ordinary people, have accomplished in life what they're going to accomplish. Or do famous people get PD because the brain, unknowingly, makes a Faustian bargain? Fame first — and then PD? Is there something about PD that leads to fame? Something that energizes the brain before slowing it down? A bi-phasic or bipolar disorder like a "slow motion-over time" form of Manic Depressive Disorder?

Dopamine and Mobility

Parkinson disease is diagnosed based on the presence of two or more of the four primary symptoms, symptoms affecting mobility: tremor, rigidity, slowness of movement, and postural instability. These symptoms mainly result from the loss of a chemical, dopamine, in a specific region of the brain — a region that regulates mobility. Dopamine facilitates the communication of cells in this region.

Disorders in mood, anxiety, and especially depression, are common in people with PD. Thus at least 40% of all people with PD are depressed. This is discussed further in Chapter 9. The depression may be a "reactive" or "external" depression; one in reaction to having PD or another external event. Or, as is more common, the depression is an "internal" or "endogenous" depression, a depression not in reaction to an outside event. In 20% of people with PD, an endogenous depression, one for no apparent reason, marks the start of PD. This is usually recognized in retrospect, after the symptoms that affect mobility have appeared. The endogenous depression of PD consists of apathy, fatigue, laziness, loss of energy, and passivity: qualities opposite to those that enabled, in a good way, Pope John Paul II and Salvador Dali, and in a bad way, Adolf Hitler.

Dopamine and Depression

What is the reason for the apathy, fatigue, laziness, loss of energy, and passivity in PD? Could these symptoms be preceded by a "mania," a surge of creative energy?

In PD, in addition to the loss of dopamine, there's a loss of cells containing two chemical cousins of dopamine, both important in regulating mood. These chemical cousins are noradrenalin (or norepinephrine) and serotonin. The noradrenalin and serotonin cells are in the brainstem near the dopamine cells. They interact with hundreds of millions of other cells, perhaps as much as 10% of the ten billion or more brain cells. A loss of dopamine, nor-adrenalin, or serotonin cells affects cells throughout the brain, resulting in changes in mood from confidence to despair, energy to fatigue, joy to depression.

The process of PD, as distinct from the recognition of PD, may begin 5, 10, or more years before the symptoms of tremor and slowed movement appear. It's possible, perhaps probable, that before depression appears, there's a stage of "excitation," a "surge of creative energy, confidence, and joy," and that's when the foundations of greatness, of fame, are laid.

The Progression of Parkinson: It Doesn't Age Like Wine

The Stages of Parkinson Disease

A frequently asked question of PD people is: "What Stage am I in?" In 1967, before Sinemet, Dr. Margaret Hoehn and Dr. Melvin Yahr created a method of rating or staging PD from 0 to 5. The stage tells you where you are today. It doesn't tell you where you'll be 1, 2, 3, 4, 5, or 10 years from now. The Hoehn and Yahr Scale is *not* a Cancer Rating Scale where the rating is a guide to treatment and outlook. The Hoehn & Yahr Scale is a limited guide to treatment and outlook. However, despite its limits, the scale has endured, attesting to its usefulness. The Hoehn & Yahr Scale, and a more detailed scale, the Unified Parkinson Disease Rating Scale (UPDRS), is used by doctors to evaluate how you are doing. Each of the scales focuses mainly on mobility. The Quality of Life Scale should be used by you to understand how you are doing. The Quality of Life Scale looks at mobility, emotions, and body functions. It complements the Hoehn and Yahr Scale.

The Hoehn & Yahr Scale

Here are the stages of the Hoehn & Yahr Scale.

0: No visible symptoms of Parkinson disease.
1: Symptoms confined to one side of the body.
2: Symptoms on both sides of the body. *No difficulty walking*
3: Symptoms on both sides of the body. *Minimal difficulty walking*
4: Symptoms on both sides of the body. *Moderate difficulty walking*
5: Symptoms on both sides of the body. *Unable to walk*

Anna, from Chapter 1, has Stage 1 Parkinson disease. Anna's symptoms affect only the right side of her body (and thus are maximum on the left or opposite side of Anna's brain). As a Stage 1 PD person, it's not surprising that Anna has a good Quality of Life. But as you'll see, mobility is only one aspect of Quality of Life. A Stage

1 PD person who is isolated, lonely, and depressed would have a bad Quality of Life if he didn't have PD. Melvin, the senator from Chapter 1, has Stage 3 PD and has a good Quality of Life. While Jack, from Chapter 2, has Stage 2 PD and has a bad Quality of Life, and Jerry, the dentist from Chapter 3, has Stage 2 PD and has a bad Quality of Life. Parkinson can change your Quality of Life — if you let it. Pope John Paul II has PD, and from newsreels showing how difficult it is for him to walk, he probably has Stage 4 PD. Yet, the Pope has an excellent Quality of Life.

Understanding and Misunderstanding the Stages of Parkinson

In 1967, the Hoehn & Yahr Scale reflected the underlying Parkinson state. Sinemet, and now Sinemet plus Comtan, have changed PD: symptoms recede or they are masked. However, no drug, as yet, halts PD's progression. Thus, when the person with PD is "staged," the staging reflects not the true stage (the underlying state of your PD), but the outward appearance. Parkinson drugs hide the true stage. This is a good thing — because in the true stage, you could not do the things you do when Sinemet is working. To find your true stage, you must be withdrawn from Sinemet or Sinemet plus Comtan for at least one month. For most people this is impossible.

After 5 years of treatment, approximately half of all people on Sinemet fluctuate. They have good and bad periods, periods when they are "on" and Sinemet is working, and periods when they are "off" and Sinemet isn't working. The off periods more closely resemble your true stage. "On and off" is discussed in Chapter 10. If you are on Sinemet and you fluctuate your doctor will stage you in an on and in an off period.

The Hoehn & Yahr Scale emphasizes walking. Among doctors, there can be debate as to what is meant by minimal difficulty walking (Stage 3 PD) and moderate difficulty walking (Stage 4 PD). Doctors rate walking while the patient strides in a straight path on level ground and look for the following:

A normal stride, where the heel of one foot clears the toe of the other foot.

A *short stride,* where the heel of one foot does not clear the toe of the other foot.
A *shuffle,* where the stride gets shorter, and shorter, until the heel of one foot no longer clears the toe of the other foot.
A *freeze,* where the stride shortens until the patient is stuck and can't move.

If while walking along a straight path you have a short stride or you shuffle, many doctors will rate you as a Stage 3 PD. If while walking you freeze one or more times and cannot recover and get going, or if you freeze and stumble, many doctors will rate you as a Stage 4 PD.

Many doctors will also rate walking while the patient turns, first to one side and then another, and will look for the following:

No difficulty while turning to the right or left.
Taking extra steps while turning to the right *or left.*
Taking extra steps while turning to the right *and left.*
Becoming stuck or "freezing" and being unable to turn to the right or left.

If you take extra steps while turning to your right or left, many doctors will rate you as Stage 3 PD (minimal difficulty). If you take extra steps while turning to your right and left, or you freeze while turning, many doctors will rate you as a Stage 4 PD (moderate difficulty). If there is a discrepancy in rating you from *when you walked in a straight path* and *when you turned,* the rating when you walked in a straight path counts. However, this isn't universally agreed upon. This explains why one doctor may rate you a Stage 3, while another doctor, seeing you at the same time, may rate you a Stage 4. Although this is infrequent, it illustrates the subjectivity of the stages.

Postural instability or difficulty maintaining balance is a primary symptom of PD. Impaired walking is a secondary symptom, not because it's less important than postural instability, but because it's made up of two symptoms: postural instability and bradykinesia.

Postural instability is responsible for falling. To test for postural instability, the doctor may walk you through the following:

> Stand with your feet together. Then he will ask:
> "Do you feel steady or unsteady?"
> Then he will have you turn to the right. Then he will ask:
> "Do you feel steady or unsteady?"
> Then he will have you turn to the left. Then he will ask:
> "Do you feel steady or unsteady?"

Being unsteady on one or more of the above indicates postural instability.

Most doctors test postural instability by asking the patient to stand with feet together. And then, from behind, the doctor holds on to each shoulder and jerks the patient backwards toward him. If the patient takes one or two steps backward, then corrects or rights himself in response to the pull postural stability is normal.

If the patient takes one or two steps backward and would fall if the doctor didn't catch him, or if the patient falls backward without taking any steps, postural stability is compromised. This is seen in Stage 3 or Stage 4 PD.

If you can't stand without falling your postural stability is markedly compromised. This is seen in Stage 5 PD. The final rating, the stage, is made by your doctor taking all the above into account.

Anna, a 62-Year-Old Woman, Five Years After Being Diagnosed with Parkinson

It's me, Anna, and I'm 5 years older and have had Parkinson for 5 more years. It's not been what I thought it would be, my fears were unfounded. Bruce, my children, and I are closer. It's our disease. We decided not to let Parkinson interfere with our lives so we traveled to China, Japan, Korea, Mongolia. We know everyone can't do it so we're grateful we could.

We stayed with the specialist at the medical center. It's more traveling, but he knows Parkinson and he's been reassuring. I know anxiety and depression take a toll, but hearing it from the specialist makes Bruce and I more determined to deal with them. Bruce and I weren't religious — but we've become so. We rejoined our support group where we discuss Parkinson, our feelings, and, since most of us are religious, we read the Bible.

I've a little more trouble turning in bed, getting up from a chair, writing, and applying make-up (I want to look alluring for Bruce). Sinemet and Comtan help — and I hardly notice the change. When I'm down, which I am, or anxious, which I am, I breathe deeply, meditate, and pray. For reassurance I call my doctor. And for more reassurance I talk to Bruce, to my family, my friends with Parkinson, and I read the Bible. I'm not on a tranquilizer or an anti-depressant. And I'm not as worried about the future. It's been a good 5 years.

I recently took the Quality of Life Exam and compar0ed it to what it was 5 years ago. My Stage 5 years ago was 1, my Stage now, on Sinemet and Comtan, is 2.

My Mobility Index on Sinemet and Comtan is 14 (out of 40 points).

My Mobility Index 5 years ago, on no medication, was 11. I know my mobility would be worse if I weren't on Sinemet and Comtan.

My Emotional Index is 9 (out of 44 points).

My Emotional Index 5 years ago was 9. If it weren't for my family, my Parkinson friends, my doctor, and the Bible, I'd be a "mental case."

My Autonomic Index is 2 (out of 16 points).

My Autonomic Index 5 years ago was 4.

It's awkward saying it, but I think Bruce and I have become closer and wiser — because of Parkinson. I like this quotation from the Book of Wisdom:

> WHERE DOES WISDOM COME FROM, WHERE IS IT FOUND?
> NO HUMAN KNOWS THE WAY TO HER, SHE IS NOT TO BE FOUND ON EARTH WHERE WE LIVE.
> "SHE IS NOT IN ME," SAYS THE ABYSS. "NOR HERE," REPLIES THE SEA.
> SHE CANNOT BE BOUGHT WITH GOLD, NOR PAID FOR WITH SILVER.
> SHE CANNOT BE SEEN BY ANY LIVING CREATURE,
> SHE IS HIDDEN FROM THE BIRDS OF THE SKY.
> DEATH AND DAMNATION BOTH SAY, "WE HAVE HEARD ONLY RUMORS OF HER."
> GOD ALONE KNOWS HER PATH.

CHAPTER

4

The Autonomic Nervous System: You Can't Live Without It

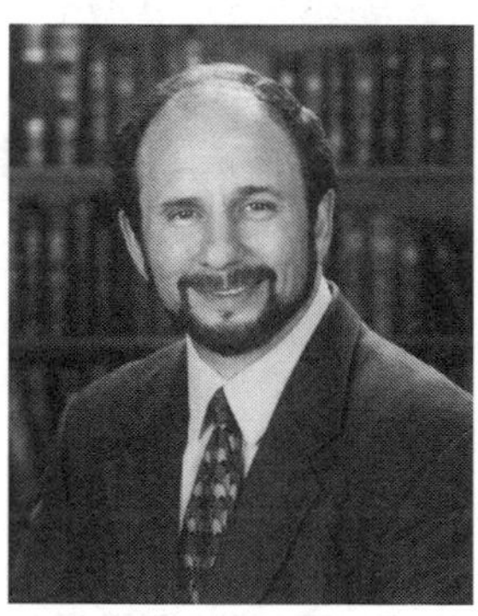

Paul Wellstone,
U.S. Senator whose father and mother suffered from PD

"I wish there had been more than family support to help my parents cope with their Parkinson disease. I wish there had been more of a community, other people dealing with Parkinson, because support from others is very important.

"I know from years of experience with my parents, and from the time I've spent with people in the Parkinson community, that those men and women who do best are men and women that have a team. It's family; it's loved ones; it's good friends; and frankly it's also other people who are dealing with this disease. There are ways in which people can be mutually supportive.

"I like to hear the words "self-reliance" and "independence" when talking about people who have PD. But you know what? I also like the word "community." I think all of us are inter-dependent and the ways in which we can support one another are really important."

The autonomic nervous system keeps people alive. It regulates body temperature, heart beat, breathing, and blood pressure. It keeps us cool in summer and warm in winter, dry in the tropics, and wet in the desert, it controls how much light enters the brain, how fast food is digested, when we go to the bathroom, it turns us on for emergencies and sex, and it calms us.

As a neurologist I've studied the autonomic nervous system for 35 years, and my wife, as an anesthesiologist, has studied it for 25 years. We've seen what it does, we're amazed, and like God, we believe in the system without fully comprehending it.

This chapter describes several ways in which the autonomic nervous system goes "haywire" in PD: in breathing, in swallowing, in digesting, in urinating, and in having sex — you can't "do it" without it. I stress the role of the autonomic nervous system in governing the body. A government so powerful and silent, that if it was in Washington, DC, the Republicans would speak of it as a "vast liberal conspiracy" and the Democrats would call it a "vast right-wing conspiracy" — both would be correct.

The Autonomic Nervous System

What is the Autonomic Nervous System?

The autonomic nervous system governs or regulates the body's internal environment. Shortly after you arrive in a doctor's office, or an emergency room, your vital signs are checked: temperature, pulse rate, blood pressure, and rate of respiration. The vital signs mirror your body's internal environment. They must be maintained for each organ: brain, heart, gut, kidneys, liver, lung, and skin to work efficiently. The autonomic nervous system does this as follows.

It maintains the body's temperature at 98.6° Fahrenheit. If the temperature rises because of an infection, a sauna, or a sun burn, the autonomic nervous system rids the body of heat by shuttling blood from the internal organs to the skin. From here the heat evaporates. As a result you feel flushed and you sweat. If you're anxious, your autonomic nervous system can be tricked into thinking your temperature is up (when it is not) causing you to feel flushed or hot.

If the body's temperature drops because of an under-active thyroid gland, or a dip in the Arctic Ocean, the autonomic nervous system warms the body by shuttling blood away from the skin to the internal organs. As a result you may feel cold or turn blue. If you're anxious your autonomic nervous system can be tricked into thinking your temperature is down (when it is not) and you may feel cold when no one else does.

The autonomic nervous system maintains the body's heart rate at between 60 and 90 beats per minute. If temperature, need for oxygen, or metabolism increases, or if the body loses body fluids (by dehydration or bleeding), or if the body is in pain, then the autonomic nervous system, through a direct line to the heart, can make it beat faster. If you're anxious, your autonomic nervous system can be tricked into making the heart beat faster and you may feel your heart pounding, feel dizzy or lightheaded, or faint.

The autonomic nervous system maintains the body's blood pressure at between 95/140 and 50/90. To maintain a stable internal environment, blood flow to critical organs must be adequate. Because flow cannot be easily measured, blood pressure is measured instead. If blood pressure falls due to standing up quickly or dehydration, blood flow to the brain decreases. For the flow to be restored the resistance of blood vessels must quickly increase. This is done by the autonomic nervous system, which increases resistance by narrowing the arteries.

If despite the narrowing, blood pressure continues to drop, flow to critical organs such as the brain, heart, and lungs is restored by shunting blood away from less critical organs such as the gut, the kidneys, the liver, or the skin. In this case the autonomic nervous system changes the resistance of the veins because 70% of circulating blood is in the veins.

If you have PD, if you are on certain PD drugs, if you're anxious, or fearful, or panicked your autonomic nervous system can be tricked into decreasing the resistance of your arteries or veins, dropping your blood pressure, making you feel dizzy, or lightheaded, or faint. This is what happens if a nurse approaches you with a large needle and syringe.

The autonomic nervous system maintains the rate of breathing below 18 breaths per minute. This stops the body from hyperventilating. If the body needs oxygen or temperature or metabolism increases, the autonomic nervous system responds by making the body breathe faster. Each breath is shallower and more energy is spent on the mechanics of breathing. This fatigues the chest muscles — the "bellows" of your lungs — making the body gasp for air.

If you're anxious and you have PD, your autonomic nervous system can be tricked into making you breathe faster or hyperventilate. When you hyperventilate, you blow off carbon dioxide. This, in turn, can make your heart pound, your vision blur, your ears ring, or make you feel dizzy, lightheaded, or faint.

The following symptoms usually, but not always, result from a disorder in the autonomic nervous system:

- Feeling your hands or feet tingling or burning.
- Feeling flushed or feverish.
- Feeling your vision is blurred.
- Feeling dizzy or lightheaded.
- Feeling that you're choking.
- Feeling that your heart is pounding.
- Feeling short of breath.
- Feeling nauseated.
- Feeling faint.
- Feeling sweaty.
- Feeling that your ears are ringing or buzzing.
- Feeling hot or cold when no one else is.

The Sympathetic Part of the Autonomic Nervous System

The sympathetic part of the autonomic nervous system starts in the hypothalamus, deep inside the brain. The hypothalamus is below the thalamus and above the pituitary or master gland. The hypothalamus governs the pituitary gland that in turn regulates:

- The thyroid gland, which regulates metabolism.
- The adrenal glands, which regulate blood pressure and fluid balance.
- The pancreas, which regulates blood sugar.
- The ovaries and testes.

The thalamus is the brain's main relay center, and through the eyes, ears, nose, and from the nerve endings in the skin, the thalamus receives information about the outside world. The thalamus also receives information about the body's internal organs from pressure sensors on the heart and large arteries; stretch sensors on the medium and small arteries and veins; pressure sensors on the major airways in the lungs; sensors in the heart, small arteries and veins, liver, kidney, and pancreas that monitor oxygen levels, blood acidity (pH), sugar, and salt concentration; and stretch sensors on the walls of the stomach, intestines, rectum, and bladder.

Information about the outside world and the internal organs, after being decoded and analyzed, is sent to your hypothalamus. Here, groups of nerve cells, called primary sympathetic cells reanalyze the information and send it to secondary sympathetic cells in the brainstem and spinal cord. Groups of secondary sympathetic cells extend along the spinal cord from the neck to the lower back. These secondary cells send information to third-order sympathetic cells located in chains that run parallel to the spinal cord. Flow of information from primary to secondary to third-order cells to their target organs is aided by the chemicals nor-adrenalin and adrenalin; on blood vessels these chemicals interact with specialized receptors.

The sympathetic nervous system can activate all of the body's organs, a few organs, or part of an organ. The fine-tuning is accomplished by activating:

- A specific number, sequence, or group of sympathetic cells.
- A specific number, sequence, or type of receptors on an organ.
- A selective release of hormones from your pituitary, thyroid, or adrenal glands, or the pancreas, ovaries or testes.

The Parasympathetic Part of the Autonomic Nervous System

The parasympathetic part of the autonomic nervous system starts in the brainstem, below the hypothalamus. Primary parasympathetic cells receive information from the outside world and your internal organs. But, compared to the sympathetic cells, the amount and quality of information is limited. After being analyzed most of it is sent via the vagus nerve to secondary parasympathetic cells located in chains near the organs they serve. Information is relayed from these cells to receptors on their target organs by the chemical acetyl-choline. The vagus serves almost every organ in the body except the rectum, bladder, uterus, and testis; these are served, via sacral nerves, by primary parasympathetic cells located in the lower spinal cord.

Despite colorful diagrams and descriptive words, the autonomic nervous system is hard to understand. Think of the sympathetic nervous system as the federal government. The federal government's central offices are in Washington, DC. Similarly, the sympathetic system's "central offices" are in the hypothalamus. The federal government has regional offices throughout the nation. Similarly, the sympathetic system's "regional offices," are on secondary cells throughout the spinal cord. The federal government has local offices in cities, counties, and towns. Similarly, the sympathetic system's "local offices" are on third-order cells near their target organs. The federal government receives feedback from its Washington, regional, local, and overseas offices and from the people and their representatives. Similarly, the sympathetic system receives information from sensors on its target organs, secondary- and third-order cells, and the thalamus.

The federal government has executive, legislative, and judicial functions. These affect you in discrete, overlapping, or, even contradictory ways. Similarly, the sympathetic system, alone or with help from one or multiple glands, can affect an organ in different or contradictory ways. Thus, if you have a bad heart it will respond to anxiety differently than if you have a normal heart.

Think of the parasympathetic part of the nervous system as a state government. There are large, populous states such as California, Texas, New York, and Florida, and less populous states such as Rhode Island, Delaware, North Dakota, and South Dakota. Each has its own capital. Similarly, the parasympathetic part of the autonomic nervous system's large populous capital offices are in the brainstem, and the less populous capital offices are in the lower spinal cord. Each state has local offices in its cities, counties, and towns. There are no regional offices. Similarly, the parasympathetic part of the autonomic nervous system's local offices are on secondary cells near their target organs. There are no third-order cells. Each state government receives feedback from its local offices, from its people and their representatives. Similarly, the parasympathetic part of the autonomic nervous system receives feedback from sensors on its target organs and their secondary cells and the thalamus. Each state has executive, legislative, and judicial functions. These affect you in discrete, overlapping, or, even contradictory ways. Similarly, the parasympathetic part of the autonomic nervous system can affect an organ in different or contradictory ways.

The federal government and the states also affect you in overlapping or even contradictory ways. Similarly, the sympathetic and parasympathetic parts of the autonomic nervous system can affect an organ or multiple organs in different or contradictory ways. Just as outside danger, disease, or pain can activate the autonomic nervous system, so too can anxiety, fear, anger and panic activate the autonomic nervous system (Figure 4.1).

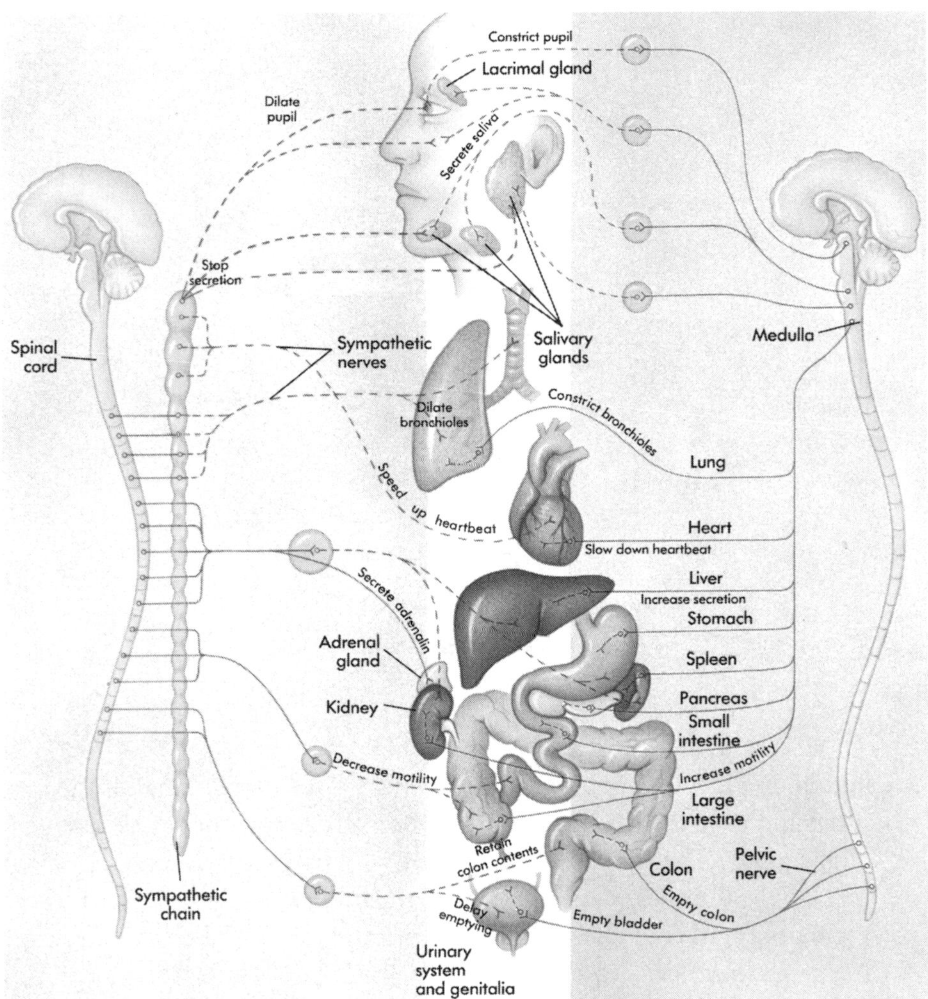

Figure 4.1 The Autonomic Nervous System

The Lungs in Parkinson Disease

How Is Breathing Regulated?

Breathing is regulated by the brainstem from a region called the respiratory center (Figure 4.2). The brainstem is located between the basal ganglia, which think about how the muscles should move, and the spinal cord, which makes the muscles move. The brainstem,

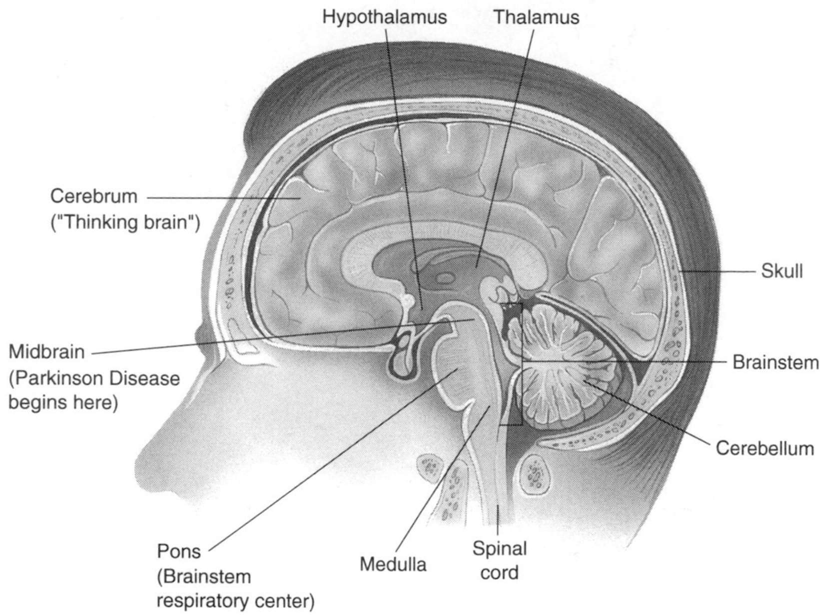

Figure 4.2 *Cerebrum-Brain in Situ*

acting, in part, through the autonomic nervous system, makes the lungs increase the rate and depth of breathing in response to specific signals. The signals include nerve signals from stretch receptors on the muscles of the chest wall, the inner-costal muscles, and the diaphragm. The chest-wall muscles and diaphragm act as a bellows, sucking air into the lungs. After the lungs extract oxygen from the air, they expel the carbon dioxide from the blood into the exhaled air. The muscles of the chest wall and diaphragm are regulated by nerve cells in the upper spinal cord. These cells are, in turn, regulated by the brainstem.

The basal ganglia, the areas of the brain affected by PD, are located above the brainstem and spinal cord. People with PD do not, because of their disease, stop breathing. However, the muscles of breathing, like the muscles in your arms and legs that are affected by PD, can become rigid and not move well. The rate of breathing is affected by anxiety. When thinking about crossing a busy street, hurrying to catch a bus, sitting in a dentist's chair waiting for a root canal, or putting out your arm to have blood drawn, your rate of breathing increases. Feeling anxious, angry, fearful, or excited calls forth energy and makes you breathe faster. When a signal is sent out from the respiratory center, the chest-wall muscles and the diaphragm, muscles that surround your lungs, contract. This increases the space between the chest wall and lungs, decreases the pressure inside the lungs (compared to that outside the body), and causes the lungs to inhale to equalize the pressure inside with that outside.

As the lungs expand to fill the space in the chest wall, a second signal is sent to relax the muscle (Figure 4.3). As the muscles relax, the space around the lungs narrows, pressure inside the lungs

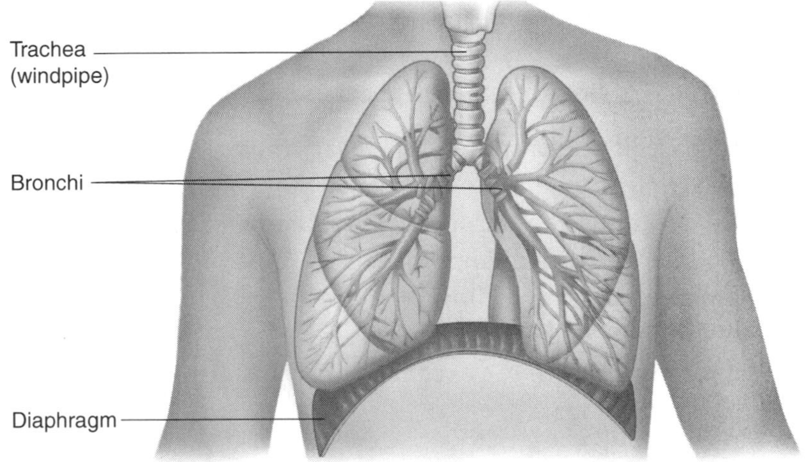

The Lungs in Parkinson Disease

1) The Lungs are encircled by 12 ribs to which are attached the 12 intercostal muscles. When the intercostal muscles expand, the lungs "suck in." When the intercostal muscles contract, they force air out of the lungs.

2) The Diaphragm moves down, expands the lungs, and "sucks in" air. The diaphragm moves up like a piston and forces air out of the lungs.

Figure 4.3 The Lungs in Parkinson Disease

increases, the lungs exhale and air is forced out. The brainstem makes its decisions regarding the rate and depth of breathing on the basis of information it receives from the body. The information includes the level of oxygen in the air, the level of oxygen in the blood, the level of expired gas and carbon monoxide in the blood, and the acidity or alkalinity of the blood. The carbon dioxide level is the single most critical factor for controlling the rate and depth of breathing. This is because the carbon dioxide level reflects the rate of energy consumption.

Conditions That Cause Shortness of Breath

Shortness of breath occurs for a variety of reasons including anxiety. If you've experienced shortness of breath, you should be aware that before shortness of breath can be attributed to anxiety, a number of conditions must be considered. A partial list appears below.

Shortness of breath can occur because of:

- Disease of one or more of the heart valves
- Heart muscle failure
- An accumulation of fluid in the sac surrounding the heart
- An altered heart rhythm
- Interference with airflow through the nose, trachea (windpipe), or bronchi (airways)
- Interference with the exchange of oxygen from the outside air to the lungs
- Diseases that restrict the movement of the lungs, such as those that cause scarring. Risk factors for such diseases include cigarette smoking and marijuana.
- Exercise that previously did not result in shortness of breath
- Lying down
- Diseases that weaken the muscles of the chest wall and diaphragm or make them rigid (such as PD)
- Diseases of the spinal cord, such as Lou Gehrig's disease and polio

- Strokes or injuries of the spinal cord, such as the injury paralyzing Christopher Reeves (Superman) and causing him to breathe with a respirator

Separating anxiety-related shortness of breath from disease-related shortness of breath may be difficult even for a skilled physician, and may often require a complete blood count and body chemistry, an arterial blood gas, a chest x-ray, an electro-cardiogram, pulmonary function tests, and an MRI. Often, anxiety-related shortness of breath accompanies or aggravates disease-related shortness of breath.

Parkinson as a Cause of Shortness of Breath

If, as a result of PD, the chest-wall muscles and diaphragm become rigid, then during inspiration they will not expand fully, and during expiration they will not relax fully. Thus, the bellows function of the lungs will be compromised. At rest, the normal rate of breathing is 12 to 18 breaths per minute. In some people with advanced PD, the rate is greater than 20 breaths per minute, causing them to spend more energy breathing, fatigue more easily, and become short of breath. Combined with heart or lung disease, or a history of smoking, these conditions will add to shortness of breath.

In PD, a severe deformity of the spine can occur, limiting the movement of the lungs and resulting in shortness of breath. While some PD people have a mild degree of deformity, a few have a deformity of sufficient severity to cause shortness of breath.

In PD, on PD drugs, dyskinesia or involuntary movements can occur. Some PD people who fluctuate on PD drugs may complain of shortness of breath. The shortness of breath can occur in an off period, before taking Sinemet, when the chest-wall muscles and diaphragm are rigid; or the shortness of breath can occur in an on period with dyskinesia, because the dyskinesia may cause the chest-wall muscles and diaphragm to contract less efficiently.

PD people with rigid chest walls, or severe spinal deformities, or severe off periods may complain of shortness of breath with exercise or when lying down. Normally when sitting or standing, gravity aids the downward movement of the diaphragm, when lying down the aid of gravity is lost. Some PD people are unable to compensate for this loss, and complain of shortness of breath. In some, the shortness of breath is so bothersome they are encouraged to sleep sitting up in a chair.

PD people, like anyone else, can be anxious, and this can result in shortness of breath. In some PD people who go off, the combination of rigidity of the chest-wall muscles and anxiety results in hyperventilation, this in turn may result in a panic attack. The treatment of panic attacks is discussed in Chapter 7.

The treatment of shortness of breath in PD starts with proper diagnosis. This may require seeing an internist, a cardiologist, and a lung specialist. If shortness of breath is not related to heart or lung disease, then shortness of breath may be related to PD. If shortness of breath is related to rigidity of the chest-wall muscles and diaphragm, additional PD medication, such as adding Comtan to Sinemet or a dopamine agonist may help. If shortness of breath is related to dyskinesia then medications should be reduced or rescheduled. General measures to reduce anxiety are discussed in Chapter 7.

Drooling in Parkinson Disease

Drooling, excess saliva, is a frequent complaint among PD people with approximately 70% complaining of it. In most people it is an annoyance consisting of a feeling of excess water in the mouth. In some, it is a major embarrassment and, potentially, a hazard because aspiration of saliva — swallowing saliva into the lungs — carries the risk of pneumonia. Saliva is a clear, watery fluid. It contains enzymes (proteins) that initiate digestion, breaking down complex sugars and starches. Saliva coats food making it slippery, helping propel it past the throat, down the esophagus (gullet), and into the stomach. If you've ever tried to swallow food when your mouth's dry you'll appreciate the role of saliva (Figure 4.4).

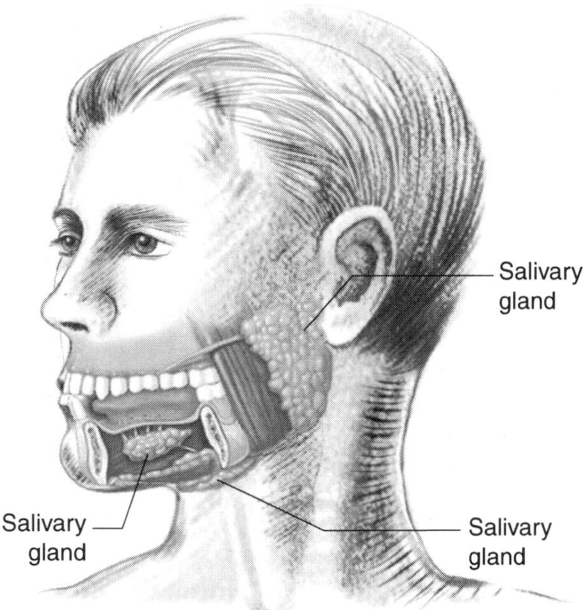

Figure 4.4 Drooling in Parkinson Disease

Drooling and Swallowing

Saliva is removed by swallowing, preventing it from accumulating in the mouth and throat and overflowing into the lungs. Swallowing is an active process that requires the coordination of the tongue and the muscles of the throat. Gravity aids swallowing. During the day, when the head is upright, while seated (or standing), saliva, propelled by the tongue and the muscles of the throat, moves down the esophagus into the stomach. The process is aided by gravity.

In PD, the muscles of the throat and esophagus are affected to varying degrees. The muscles become rigid and lose, in part, their ability to encircle, massage, and propel food down the esophagus and into the stomach. This usually (but not always) occurs late in PD. Any process that reduces the ability to swallow food, reduces the ability to swallow saliva. Saliva is mainly produced by the parotid glands, egg-like bodies in the floor of the mouth at the angle of your jaw.

The Dynamics of Drooling

Saliva is produced throughout the day and night. Although the production of saliva is automatic, its production can be increased (or less frequently decreased) in response to outside events. The sight of food, the smell of food, the taste of food, even the thought of food, automatically increases the production and flow of saliva. The sight of food or the chewing of food can make you drool. The production of saliva is under the control of the autonomic nervous system. Specialized nerve fibers originate from parasympathetic cells in the lower brainstem. The process (as yet unknown) that causes PD also affects these parasympathetic cells. In general, the parasympathetic and sympathetic parts of the autonomic nervous system oppose each other acting as brakes and accelerators. The braking and accelerating actions differ from organ to organ. Stimulation of the parasympathetic system increases salivation. Stimulation of the sympathetic system may decrease salivation. Nerve impulses from parasympathetic (or sympathetic) cells are carried down parasympathetic (or sympathetic) nerves to the vicinity of a particular organ, such as your parotid gland. Here the nerve impulses release a chemical. The chemical is stored in the terminal part of the nerve. In the parasympathetic nerve the chemical is acetyl-choline.

In general, but not always, drugs that block the parasympathetic system result, by default, in stimulation of the sympathetic system. And in general, but not always, drugs that stimulate the parasympathetic system result in blockade of the sympathetic system. Similar effects on the parasympathetic system result from drugs that block or stimulate the sympathetic system. The presence of two parallel systems, the parasympathetic and sympathetic, with usually (but not always) opposite effects on an organ and with usually (but not always) opposite responses to a particular drug, often make it difficult to predict how a particular drug will affect a particular organ. Especially when both systems, the parasympathetic and sympathetic, have been affected by PD.

Why Drool?

Drooling in PD results from an inability to swallow saliva. This results from rigidity and reduced mobility of the muscles of the throat and esophagus. Initially only one set of muscles may be rigid: usually the muscles of the throat. Eventually, as PD advances, the muscles of the esophagus become rigid. Rarely, drooling results from an over-production of saliva. Evidence that drooling mainly results from reduced swallowing comes from a study in which doctors measured saliva production in 83 PD people and 65 similarly aged controls. Saliva production in PD was 36% less than controls. Yet, PD people drooled and controls didn't. Thus, the doctors concluded that drooling in PD results from reduced swallowing.

Early in PD, people may experience difficulty in swallowing saliva as wetness of the pillow. During the day, with the head up, gravity compensates for any difficulty in swallowing saliva. At night, with the head down, gravity no longer compensates and saliva drips onto the pillow. This is more likely to happen when sleeping on the stomach (face down). In some people, the difficulty swallowing saliva at night is marked, as they cough, choke, or regurgitate their saliva. Such people may be forced to sleep upright, sitting in a chair.

Is Drooling Serious?

Drooling, if it occurs, is awkward, an embarrassment, not a hazard. But in people with advanced PD, drooling is not an embarrassment, it is a hazard. Such people may aspirate, swallowing saliva into their lungs, causing pneumonia. People with marked rigidity of the muscles of the throat include people with advanced PD and people with PD-like disease such as Shy Drager (discussed in Chapter 5).

People with excessive daytime drooling (drooling while the head is upright) usually, but not always, have obvious difficulty swallowing food. They usually, but not always, have difficulty speaking. The difficulty is with the physical act of speaking as distinct from the intellectual act of formulating speech. The difficulty speaking involves the muscles of the throat, larynx (voice box), muscles of breathing, and may involve the lips and tongue. The muscles that help with speaking are the same as the muscles that help with swallowing. In PD, speaking and swallowing may both be affected. But since speaking involves a different combination and sequence of these muscles, speaking can be affected without swallowing and vice versa.

Drooling can be embarrassingly obvious as you hold a handkerchief or a paper towel to your mouth. Moreover, to the general public, drooling is associated (erroneously) with mental retardation. Thus a PD person who drools not only has to contend with his disease, but with the perception that he is mentally retarded.

The Treatment of Drooling

The first approach to treating drooling is educational. The reasons for drooling are explained and you're taught to cope. You're taught to sleep (or rest) with your head upright, and to chew food slowly and carefully, swallowing frequently. These hints are helpful but eventually, as PD progresses, become unsatisfactory. A simple approach is chewing gum or sucking hard candy. This over-rides the automatic act of swallowing, by a conscious act. This is the same as forcing yourself to swing your arm or take a longer step while walking. Chewing gum is helpful in situations where drooling is embarrassing.

A second approach is prescribing PD drugs such as Sinemet plus Comtan or a dopamine agonist to improve swallowing. The drugs have limited usefulness having to do with the make-up of the muscles. The skeletal or voluntary muscles, the visible muscles of your arms and legs, are different from the involuntary muscles, the internal or smooth muscles of the throat, esophagus, trachea, bronchial tubes, bowels, and bladder. Skeletal muscles are striated or striped. When examined under a microscope they appear striped (they have striations from the Latin word for *striped*). Striated muscles are organized as individual cells, each cell connected by a motor nerve to a motor nerve cell in the spinal cord. Communication between the spinal cord and the muscle is facilitated by acetyl-choline.

Smooth muscles are not striped. Smooth muscles are organized as interconnected cell groups. In striated muscles there's point-to-point contact: one motor nerve fiber releasing a burst of acetyl-choline that excites a single receptor on a single striated muscle cell. In smooth muscle there is no point-to-point contact: multiple parasympathetic fibers releasing multiple bursts of acetyl-choline that excite multiple receptors on multiple interconnected smooth muscle cells. In addition, in smooth muscles, the actions of acetyl-choline are opposed by the actions of noradrenaline (secreted by sympathetic nerve cells). In PD a decrease in dopamine cells in the brainstem results in rigidity and slowness of the striated muscles. Restoring dopamine with Sinemet plus Comtan decreases the rigidity and increases the speed of striated muscles. The brainstem dopamine cells do not affect the smooth muscles as much as the striated muscles. The improvement in swallowing from Sinemet plus Comtan results from the actions of dopamine on bands of striated muscle in the throat and upper esophagus.

A third approach is anticholinergic drugs. The anticholinergic drugs are synthetic compounds related to belladonna. Belladonna blocks the actions of acetyl-choline at acetyl-choline receptors in the brain, on parasympathetic nerves (inside and outside the brain), and on smooth muscles and selected glands, including the parotid. Belladonna has little effect on acetyl-choline receptors on striated muscles. Some anticholinergic drugs are more specific for one group of receptors than another. Some anticholinergic drugs enter the brain, some (such as Robinul) don't. In the brain acetyl-choline opposes the actions of dopamine and drugs that block acetyl-choline increase the actions of dopamine. The anticholinergic drugs are less effective than Sinemet. As a bonus the anticholinergic drugs block the actions of acetyl-choline in the parotid gland thus decreasing drooling.

Few people with PD can tolerate doses of anticholinergic drugs high enough to stop drooling without side effects. Acetyl-choline in the brain is essential for normal intellectual function. People 60 years and older, which includes most PD people, are more sensitive to acetyl-choline than younger people. By blocking acetyl-choline inside the brain, the anticholinergic drugs can result in agitation, delusions, hallucinations, and memory loss. By blocking the actions of acetyl-choline outside the brain, the anticholinergic drugs can, in addition to having the desirable effect of decreasing drooling, have the undesirable effect of aggravating constipation.

Charcot, the great 19th-century French neurologist and teacher of Sigmund Freud, discovered the actions of belladonna. Parisian women of the 19th century used belladonna eye drops to dilate their pupils — making them appear more attractive, more seductive. However, in dilating their pupils, their vision became blurred. At a reception, a Parisian beauty may have bumped into Charcot. Learning who he was she complained of the price she paid for being alluring: blurred vision, a rapid heartbeat — and a dry mouth. Good manners precluded her from mentioning constipation. Charcot, being ignorant of acetyl-choline receptors (they weren't discovered till the 20th century), but knowing his PD people drooled, got the idea of treating them with belladonna.

Detrol, an anticholinergic drug with selective action on the wall of the bladder and few of the traditional anticholinergic side effects, can help some people control drooling. The dose is 2 mg one hour before a social situation.

A fourth approach is botulinum toxin. Anticholinergic drugs rarely affect one set of receptors, such as the parotid glands, without affecting other receptors. Because anticholinergic drugs are small molecules, they diffuse from their site of administration, gain access to the circulation and appear everywhere. Botulinum toxin is a large protein molecule that blocks acetyl-choline. Because it is a large molecule, it is difficult for botulinum toxin to go anywhere. Thus the effects of botulinum toxin remain confined to its site of injection.

Botulinum toxin is purified from bacterial cultures of clostridium botulinum and is a potent biological poison (or toxin). Clostridium botulinum, if it invades the body, breaches the body's defenses, multiplies, and if its toxin gets into the circulation, can result in botulism. Botulism, unrecognized and untreated, is fatal. The toxin, when properly administered by a trained specialist is safe. The toxin doesn't leave the injection site, because there is no living bacteria to multiply, there is nothing to produce more toxin. The activity of botulinum toxin is measured in mouse-units. A mouse-unit is the amount of toxin needed to kill 50% of a group of mice by injecting the toxin into the intra-peritoneal space (the space surrounding the gut). Injecting the toxin into the intra-peritoneal space guarantees the toxin will get into the circulation. Botulinum toxin, when injected into a striated muscle, causes paralysis of the muscle by stopping the release of acetyl-choline from the nerve endings onto the muscle.

Two types of toxin are available: A and B. Both are approved for use in conditions that are characterized by local spasm (dystonia) of striated muscles. These conditions include forced eye-lid closure (blepharospasm). In recent studies 25 to 50 mouse-units of botulinum toxin was injected into each parotid gland. Care was taken to avoid injecting the toxin into the floor of the mouth. Such an injection could weaken the muscles of the mouth and affect swallowing. Preliminary results indicate that injections of botulinum decrease drooling for weeks and are a good way to stop drooling.

Swallowing in Parkinson Disease

The articles on swallowing, the stomach, and constipation in PD, were adapted, in part, from articles written for the *NPF Parkinson Report* by Dr. Ron Pfeiffer of the University of Tennessee.

How Many People with Parkinson Have Difficulty Swallowing?

Depending on how the question is asked, 30% to 95% of people with PD say they have difficulty swallowing. In most the difficulty is minor, in some it is major. If swallowing is tested, 75% to 95% of people with PD have difficulty. In most the difficulty is minor and they're not aware of it.

The Dynamics of Swallowing

Swallowing requires the coordinated action of many muscles both striated and smooth. (See Figure 2.1 on page 27.) First the tongue and jaw muscles prepare the food to be swallowed by chewing it and mixing it with saliva. Next, the muscles in the back of the mouth and throat (the pharyngeal muscles) start to swallow. They also seal off the windpipe and nose to keep food and liquids from backing up into them. Next, the muscles of the esophagus propel the food into the stomach. Slow or rigid muscles, at any level can result in difficulty swallowing. The same slowness and rigidity that affects the muscles in the arms and legs affects the muscles in the throat. A serious complication of difficulty swallowing is aspiration pneumonia. About 25% of people with PD at one time or another aspirate. In many aspiration is announced by coughing or choking. In some it is silent. Difficulty swallowing may result in marked and unintentional weight loss.

The Treatment of Swallowing

Treating the primary symptoms of PD: rigidity and slowness by increasing or adjusting Sinemet plus Comtan, the dopamine agonists, or the anticholinergic drugs is helpful in 50% of people. Detrol, which is helpful in drooling, may be helpful in swallowing. Training sessions with speech and swallowing therapists are also helpful. In a small group of people with PD, perhaps 5%, abnormal muscle bands may partly block swallowing, or pouches may form, trapping food. In these people, identified by a barium swallow, surgery may correct the difficulty.

The Swallowing Questionnaire

If you have difficulty swallowing, complete the Swallowing Questionnaire and discuss it with your doctor. The tips following the table may improve your swallowing.

THE SWALLOWING QUESTIONNAIRE

Read the following statements and circle yes or no.

1.	I've lost weight recently.	Yes	No
2.	I drool.	Yes	No
3.	I cough when I eat or drink.	Yes	No
4.	I choke when I eat or drink.	Yes	No
5.	I have heartburn.	Yes	No
6.	I have difficulty propelling food to the back of my mouth.	Yes	No
7.	I have difficulty keeping food or liquids in my mouth.	Yes	No
8.	It takes me a long time to finish eating.	Yes	No
9.	I feel food sticks in my throat.	Yes	No
10.	I have difficulty swallowing pills.	Yes	No

- Take small bites.
- Swallow twice after every bite.
- Take small sips.
- Alternate bites and sips; this clears the food from your mouth.
- Don't talk with food in your mouth.
- Keep your chin parallel to the table. If your chin's too far down, you can't keep food in your mouth. People with PD may, without knowing it, bend their necks, forcing their chins down. This makes chewing (and swallowing) difficult. Bend your neck so your eyes look at the floor. Now try to chew. It's difficult because by bending your neck you put your jaw muscles at a mechanical disadvantage. Now raise your neck so your eyes look 30 degrees above the horizontal. Now try to chew. It's easy because your jaw muscles are at a mechanical advantage. Because you can't always remind yourself to raise your chin, I tell people with PD to sit with their elbows on the table; this automatically raises their chin, and helps chewing and swallowing.
- Change your diet. Certain foods such as raw vegetables, nuts, and peanut butter may be difficult to swallow and should be avoided. A swallowing therapist or a dietitian can recommend foods that are easy to swallow.

The Stomach in Parkinson Disease

The stomach is a hollow tube made-up of smooth muscle and acid-secreting glands (Figure 4.5). The smooth muscles encircle the stomach and "massage" food from it into the intestines. In normal aging the smooth muscles lose their tone, the stomach becomes "lax," food accumulates and does not pass easily into the intestines. This is accelerated in PD and accounts, in part, for symptoms such as bloating, burping, distention, fullness, and nausea that follow eating. This laxness, or stomach bradykinesia, can reduce the effectiveness of Sinemet. To reach the bloodstream (and ultimately the brain) Sinemet must pass through the stomach intact into the small intestine. Here the levodopa in Sinemet is absorbed into the blood. If Sinemet is held up in the stomach, enzymes change levodopa to dopamine. Because dopamine cannot enter the brain, this effectively reduces the dose of Sinemet you swallowed. Moreover, the dopamine that's formed excites dopamine receptors in the stomach. This further delays emptying of the stomach, allowing more levodopa to be changed to dopamine, further reducing the dose of Sinemet. This may account, in part, for the "wearing off" and "on off" effect (see Chapter 10).

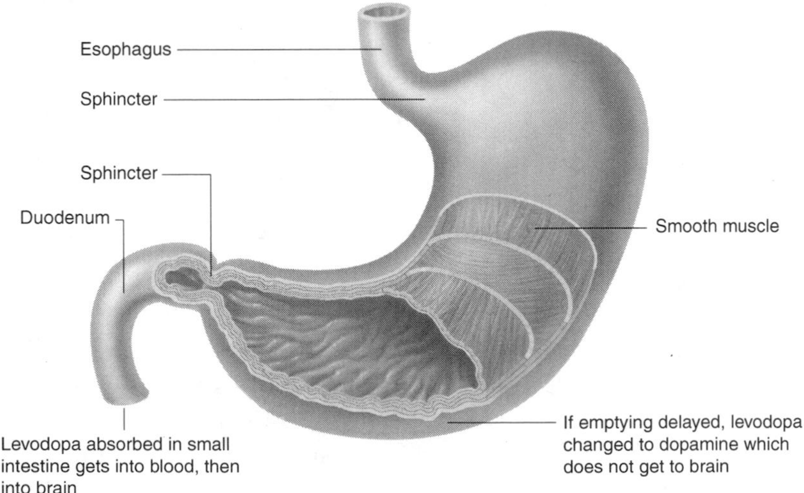
Esophagus
Sphincter
Sphincter
Duodenum
Smooth muscle
Levodopa absorbed in small intestine gets into blood, then into brain
If emptying delayed, levodopa changed to dopamine which does not get to brain

***Figure 4.5** The Stomach in Parkinson Disease*

The treatment of stomach bradykinesia in PD is similar to its treatment in other diseases such as diabetes. Because dopamine in the stomach delays emptying, drugs that block dopamine improve emptying. Metoclopramide (Reglan) is such a drug. However, Reglan gets into the brain where it blocks dopamine and worsens PD. If you have PD, you should not take Reglan. Domperidone (Motilium) blocks stomach dopamine. But as it does not get into the brain it can be used in PD. Domperidone is not marketed in the United States but can be easily and legally obtained from Canada, Europe, and Mexico (go to *www.parkinson.org*). Another drug cisapride (Propulsid), which works independently of dopamine, is also helpful. But its use is restricted because of potential heart problems.

Constipation

What Is Constipation?

Constipation is a frequent symptom of PD. Lack of a daily bowel movement isn't constipation, in fact, three bowel movements per week is normal. Constipation may be defined as two or fewer bowel movements per week. In studying constipation doctors measure the "colon transit time," which is at least twice as long in people with PD, with or without constipation, as in comparably aged people. Decreased frequency of bowel movements, two or fewer per week, occurs in 30% of people with PD. However, difficulty completing a bowel movement, with straining and incomplete evacuation (difficulty defecating) is more common, occurring in 70% of people with PD. Many people have both constipation and difficulty defecating; it is important to distinguish between these two problems because their treatments differ. In some people with PD, perhaps 5%, constipation and difficulty defecating results in fecal impaction, bloating, discomfort, and pain. It is diagnosed by a rectal examination. Usually, the impaction has to be removed manually. Proper bowel habits can prevent impaction.

Why People with Parkinson Are Constipated

Normally the muscles of the bowel wall propel stool forward. However, the rigidity and slowness that affects other muscles can affect the bowels, called bradykinesia of the bowel. Because the bowels move slowly, stool moves slowly, and the fluid that's mixed in with the stool dries out, making the stool hard. The longer the stool takes to pass through the bowel, the harder it becomes, and the more difficult it becomes to pass.

The bowels are regulated in part by the parasympathetic nervous system. However, this is only part of the picture. The bowels have their own nervous system, called the enteric nervous system, a cousin to the autonomic nervous system. If the sympathetic nervous system is like the federal government, and the parasympathetic nervous system is like a state government, then the enteric nervous system is like a large city government — a New York, or Los Angeles, or Chicago, or Miami, a government with a mind of its own. There are at least 2 million nerve cells in the enteric nervous system, as many as in the spinal cord. This may explain why drugs have such inconsistent effects on bowel function. While the cause of constipation is assumed to be a loss of brain dopamine, it may, instead, result from a loss of enteric nervous system dopamine. The loss of dopamine in the brain or in the enteric nervous system causes the bowels to move slowly.

Difficulty in Defecating Is Different from Constipation

To defecate, the muscles of the stomach must squeeze down, the muscles of the pelvis must relax, the muscles encircling the colon and anus must squeeze out stool, and the anal sphincter must open (Figure 4.6). A lack of coordination among these muscles coupled with rigidity and slowness results in difficulty defecating. Before assuming difficulty results from PD, conditions such as polyps, tumors, and diverticulitis must be ruled out. An evaluation should include a rectal exam, a proctoscopy or sigmoidoscopy, and, if necessary, a colonoscopy.

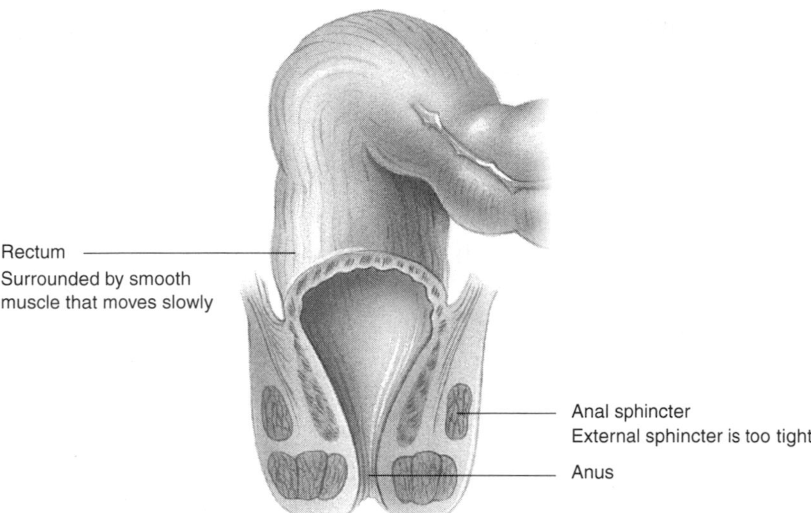

Figure 4.6 *The Rectum in Parkinson Disease*

The Treatment of Constipation

This article was adapted, in part, from one written for the NPF, by Kathrynne Holden MS, RD, an expert nutritionist.

First is fiber. As your colon transit time slows, water is absorbed from your stool making it hard. Fiber, in addition to cleansing your bowel, acts like sawdust soaking up water, allowing it to remain in your stool, preventing your stool from drying out and becoming hard. In a study where dietary fiber intake was estimated in PD people it was found that the average fiber intake was only two-thirds of the recommended daily dose of 20 grams. Increased dietary fiber then is the first step and is achieved by eating fiber-rich foods such as fruits including dates, figs, and prunes; vegetables; unprocessed bran cereal; whole grains; and beans, such as fava and kidney beans. Fava beans as a bonus contain levodopa. A six-ounce serving of fava beans may be the equal of 250 mg of levodopa. Dietary fiber can be supplemented with methyl cellulose (Citrucel), psyllium (Metamucil), or polycarbophil (FiberCon or Fiberall). With this approach you should drink six to eight glasses of water a day.

Second is regular exercise to strengthen the muscles of your abdomen and pelvis. Walking promotes movement of stool into your colon and rectum.

Third is a stool softener such as Colace.

Fourth is *senna paste,* a folk remedy. Take a four-ounce package of senna tea (senna tea is a traditional medicinal called Smooth Move). Put the senna tea in three cups of boiling water; steep for five minutes. Add the senna tea to a large pot. Next, add one pound pitted prunes, one pound raisins, one pound figs. Boil tea and fruit for five minutes. Remove from heat and let cool. Add one cup of lemon juice. Use a blender to mix to a smooth paste. Place in a glass container and store in the freezer. Paste will not freeze, and will keep for a long time. Use one or two tablespoons daily. This can be done several ways, including spreading it on toast.

Fifth is laxatives. Start with lactulose, or sorbital, or GoLytely, a glycol solution, used to clean the bowels before colonoscopy. Enemas or irritant laxatives, such as bisacodyl, cascara, or magnesia are last resorts.

The Treatment of Difficulty Defecating

Treatment for constipation may not help defecation and sometimes may make things worse by increasing the need to have a bowel movement without improving the ability to do so. There is evidence that PD people, when they're in an off period when Sinemet isn't working, have more difficulty defecating than when they're on and Sinemet is working. Adding Comtan to Sinemet by increasing on time may help defecation by improving rectal-muscle function.

Recognizing that slowed or inappropriate closing of the anal sphincter might, in part, be responsible for difficulty defecating has led some doctors to inject the anal sphincter with botulinum toxin. But this must be used with caution, as a lax sphincter is as bad as a tight sphincter.

The Bladder in Parkinson Disease

This article was adapted from one written for the NPF Parkinson Report *by Dr. Carlos Singer of the University of Miami.*

The Dynamics of the Bladder

The normal process of bladder filling proceeds silently as the bladder's walls become distended (Figure 4.7). You aren't aware of the process until the contents reach 1,000 ml or one liter (about one quart). At this time, the bladder starts signaling the brain that the time for voiding has arrived. The brain, now aware of what's happening, stops the bladder from voiding until an appropriate time. Once all is ready, the brain gives the go-ahead and the bladder contracts while at the same time the bladder sphincter opens.

A network of brain cells including the basal ganglia and the autonomic nervous system ensures the timing is synchronized. The basal ganglia allow the brain to stop the bladder from contracting while it fills. In PD, as the basal ganglia are changed, the bladder contracts prematurely in the presence of much less than 1,000 ml of urine. This is called an irritable or spastic bladder, or detrusor hyperreflexia for the muscle that contracts the bladder wall. Such premature contractions are not strong enough to empty the bladder, but

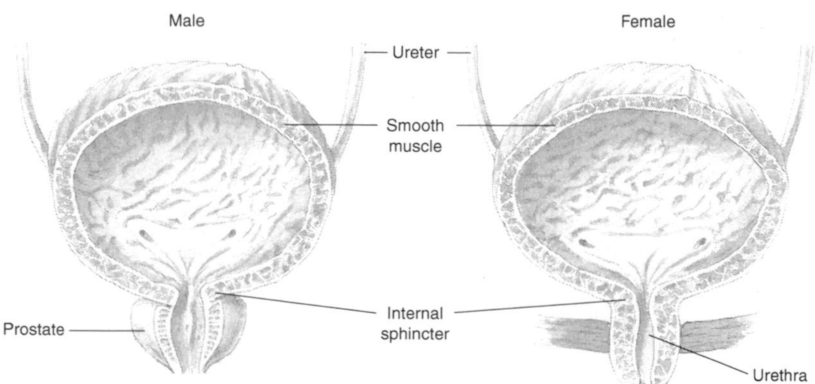

Figure 4.7 *The Bladder in Parkinson Disease*

they send enough signals to the brain to create a sense of urgency, a sensation that a person without PD may only feel if he (or she) hasn't emptied his (or her) bladder for several hours. The PD person rushes to the bathroom only to empty a small amount of urine. Since the process, called urinary frequency, repeats itself, the visits to the bathroom become more numerous both during the day and at night (nocturia). Remember, urgency can be caused by a diuretic (water pill) prescribed to prevent swelling in the feet or to control blood pressure. And urgency may result from all the water you were told to drink to relieve your constipation. If these are causing urgency, and urgency comes at times that are embarrassing, timing of the water pill and the drinking of the extra water can be re-arranged.

Urinary urgency can become so strong that if the PD person, already troubled by slowness of movement, fails to reach a bathroom on time, he (or she) has an accident, sometimes called urge incontinence. Some PD people complain of strain during urination, also called hesitancy, and of a weak stream. These symptoms suggest obstruction to the flow of urine by an enlarged prostate or a scarred bladder neck. Whereas people with PD may complain of urgency and frequency, and rarely be unable to void, people with Multiple System Atrophy, a PD-like disease, are more often unable to void.

Evaluating the Bladder

If a PD person develops these symptoms, they should not assume they are a result of PD. They should ask the doctor. If the doctor thinks it is advisable, he or she will recommend a urologist. The urologist will do a urine analysis, to exclude an infection of the bladder, and an examination of the prostate (for men) or of the bladder neck (for women). Enlargement of the prostate or scarring of the bladder neck may cause premature bladder contractions. As part of the evaluation the urologist will do urodynamics. Here, the bladder is slowly filled with saline and premature contractions are detected by special sensors. If an enlarged prostate or scarred bladder neck are found, then surgery is recommended. Symptoms may not result from an enlarged prostate or a scarred bladder neck, but from PD. And the surgery, even when done correctly and without complications, may not cure symptoms. Presently, the best and most experienced urologist cannot distinguish prostate or bladder neck urgency from PD urgency. Surgery may well be indicated but the desired result may not be attained and further measures may be necessary.

The Treatment of Urgency, Frequency, and Hesitancy

If a cause for surgery isn't found, or if symptoms continue after surgery, the urologist may prescribe drugs to relax the bladder. Detrol and Ditropan are helpful. Ditropan, an anticholinergic drug, blocks a set of nerves that carries messages to the bladder muscles and the bladder's sphincter. Detrol, also an anticholinergic drug, is more specific, it blocks mainly the bladder muscles and has fewer side effects. Detrol and Ditropan, like other anticholinergics, may cause dryness of the mouth and constipation. If you have glaucoma, you should tell the doctor before he prescribes Detrol or Ditropan. There are differences in the actions of anticholinergic drugs, and unlike drugs such as Artane, Akineton, Cogentin, and Kemardrin (anticholinergic drugs used to treat the symptoms of PD), Detrol and Ditropan are unlikely to cause the bladder to go into retention, resulting in an inability to void.

Cardura and Hytrin are not anticholinergic drugs. They relax smooth muscles including those of the bladder. They are used to treat enlarged prostate glands (by relaxing the smooth muscle of the gland) and high blood pressure (by relaxing the smooth muscle of the blood vessels). Since they lower blood pressure, you must be careful when standing up as your blood pressure may drop rapidly and you could feel dizzy. Cardura and Hytrin are also used to treat the urgency and frequency of PD. All of the drugs that relax smooth muscle can, to different degrees, weaken bladder contractions and cause retention. This is more likely in the presence of diseases such as diabetes that weaken the bladder.

Some PD people experience a delay in relaxing the sphincter at the time they void because the effects of Sinemet wear off. This can be helped by adding Comtan to each dose of Sinemet.

The Treatment of Incontinence

Urinary incontinence, uncontrolled or inappropriate urination, is an embarrassing symptom. Some people with PD are incontinent because they can't get to the bathroom in time. Some PD women are incontinent because of a relaxed pelvic floor secondary to child bearing. Some PD men are incontinent because of complications of prostate surgery. And some people with PD are incontinent because of dementia — they go when they want to go whether it is appropriate or not. The following tips are helpful with incontinence:

- Wear pull-up pants rather than those with buttons or zippers.
- Empty your bladder completely. Many people don't realize they still have urine in their bladder after voiding because the urge is gone. Remain at the toilet for an extra minute and try to void again.
- Wear undergarments made for incontinence. They have an absorbent core that keeps your skin dry, preventing irritation and eliminating odor.
- If you are a woman, do Kegel exercises to strengthen the muscles of the pelvic floor, the muscles that control urinary leakage. To do Kegel exercises, pretend you're stopping the flow of urine. You'll feel these muscles tense. Then relax. Do 20 Kegel exercises each time you have an accident.

Sex and Parkinson Disease

The Human Sexual Response

There are four phases of the human sexual response.

1. Excitement or arousal
2. Plateau
3. Orgasm
4. Resolution

Arousal can be triggered by a limitless array of thoughts, emotions, and sensations from listening to romantic music, to dining under candle light, to viewing an erotic film. During arousal, the sympathetic part of the autonomic nervous system is activated and the heart beats faster, blood pressure rises, lungs breathe harder, the body feels warm, and the genitals fill with blood, becoming engorged and growing in size. In men, an erection appears, in women their clitoris enlarges, their vagina is lubricated and swells. There's a gradual buildup of muscle tension throughout the body.

During plateau, erection, swelling, lubrication, and muscular tension reach peak levels. When orgasm occurs there's a dramatic release in tension through ejaculation in men and vaginal contraction in women. In resolution, as the sympathetic nervous system is turned off, the body returns to its pre-arousal state.

Age, Sex, and Parkinson

As people age, whether or not they have PD, it takes longer to become aroused, reach orgasm, and become excited a second time. And everyone has periods when they are not in the mood. This can be caused by many things including anxiety, depression, fatigue, overwork, and loss of self-esteem. All of these can be present in the person with PD in addition to features unique to PD. Thus some aspects of your appearance, such as a tremor, may cause you to be embarrassed or lose self-esteem. Drooling may make you think you're less attractive to your partner. If relevant this must be discussed and resolved.

Some PD people, because of their physical limitations, no longer maintain proper grooming. Thus, hair may grow from the nose or ears and teeth may not be clean. If relevant, this should be corrected. If you move slowly or have difficulty turning in bed, you may be unable to perform. Using satin bed sheets or wearing satin night garments can facilitate turning toward and onto your partner. Taking Sinemet plus Comtan, or a dopamine agonist one hour before going to bed can improve mobility and performance in bed.

Do Not Let Parkinson Kill Romance

Desire precedes arousal and without desire there's no arousal. If the PD person is not aroused by their partner, but is aroused by pornographic movies, magazines, or other partners, then there's a problem unrelated to PD. Partners should be sympathetic, but, in turn, the unaroused person must make an effort comparable to the one made on their wedding night. Your partner should be aware of the problems unique to people with PD. This includes a decreased sense of smell, resulting in an inability to be aroused by provocative perfumes, hair oils, and body parts. Visual stimuli are more effective. Which ones? Anything that works. And caress, hug, or hold each other because it is the greatest turn on you can share. Always communicate your desires to your partner, and ask your partner, in return, to communicate their desires to you.

Folk Remedies to Put You in the Mood

Folk remedies have, from antiquity, been used to put people in the mood. While their success hasn't been subjected to double-blind studies, their lore never fails to fascinate. Folk remedies include: absinthe, ambergris, animal testes, basil, cannabis, caraway, caviar, clams, coriander, crayfish, cumin, dill, eels, endives, fennel, figs, garlic, ginger, ginseng, juniper, mint, mushrooms, mustard, nutmeg, onions, paprika, prawns, quince, radishes, sesame, snails, shallots, snuff, squid, tarragon, thyme, truffles, and vitamin E. These remedies are not recommended.

Can Hormones Put You in the Mood?

Diabetes, an underactive or an overactive thyroid gland, an underactive adrenal gland, an underactive pituitary gland, a specific type of hormone-secreting tumor of the pituitary gland, or an underactive pair of testicles or ovaries, can dampen desire and block arousal in men and women. If suspected, these conditions can be tested for and corrected. If you're a man, a modest deficiency of testosterone will result in decreased beard formation, small testicles, lack of desire, and impotence, alerting you and your doctor. However, a minor deficiency of testosterone may result in lack of desire or impotence without other symptoms. If there's doubt as to whether a deficiency of testosterone is causing your lack of desire or impotence, a trial of testosterone (one month or less) may be indicated.

Are Bad Arteries Keeping You from Being Aroused?

Lack of arousal, the ability to achieve a penile or clitoral erection, as distinct from a lack of desire, may be caused by disease of the large arteries, including the arteries to the pelvis, groin, and legs. Disease of the large arteries is accelerated by smoking, diabetes, high-blood pressure, and high cholesterol. Lack of arousal may also be caused by disease of the small arteries and veins. It is well documented in men, and less in women, that disease of the arteries results in difficulty in getting an erection while disease of the veins results in difficulty in keeping an erection. Disease of the veins results in failure to keep a penile or clitoral erection because the veins can't constrict. After an erection is achieved, blood normally leaks from the erectile tissue back into the veins. To preserve an erection, the veins constrict, preventing blood from leaking. The signal for the veins to constrict comes from the autonomic nervous system.

In disease of the arteries or veins position is important. Certain positions may promote filling of the arteries and prevent draining of the veins, resulting in a prolonged and satisfying erection. Each couple should explore different positions and find the ones most satisfactory to them.

Are Drugs Keeping You from Being Aroused?

Alcohol, in moderation, by repressing social inhibitions, can increase desire and arousal. In excess, alcohol can result, temporarily, in a lack of desire and arousal. Some drugs that lower high blood pressure may reduce arousal. The lack of arousal may be related or unrelated to the drop in blood pressure. As a rule, drugs that lower blood pressure by acting on the receptors of the autonomic nervous system, drugs such as alpha blockers or beta-blockers are more likely to reduce arousal than drugs acting on calcium channels or on the angiotensin-converting enzymes. Some drugs such as phentolamine, by relaxing the arteries, increase arousal. The commonly used PD drugs, such as Sinemet plus Comtan, selegiline, Mirapex, Permax, or Requip, rarely block or reduce arousal. PD drugs that may block arousal include the anticholinergic drugs, the tricyclic anti-depression drugs, and beta-blockers.

As a rule if a lack of penile or clitoral arousal occurs within a few days or a month of starting a drug, the drug must be considered as being guilty. Almost any drug, prescription or non-prescription, whether obtained in a pharmacy or health food store, may reduce or block arousal. If a drug reduces arousal, stopping the drug invariably helps.

Arousal and the Autonomic Nervous System

Among people with PD the main cause of reduced arousal is a faulty autonomic nervous system. The autonomic nervous system sends messages to the lower spinal cord, which in turn sends them to the penis and testes, or vagina and clitoris. People with PD are usually able to be aroused. This reflects an adequate flow of blood from the arteries to the penis or clitoris, with appropriate filling and hardening of the erectile tissue. However, the PD person is unable to stay aroused. This reflects a failure of the autonomic nervous system to constrict the veins surrounding the erectile tissue, resulting in a leak back into the circulation, with penile or clitoral softening. In the presence of advanced autonomic nervous system disease as with Lenny in Chapter 5 who has Shy-Drager Syndrome, or with the use of some drugs, failure of the veins to constrict is associated with failure of the arteries to fill, so, although the desire to have sex may be present, you may be unable to perform.

So Why Can't I Become Aroused?

If you have the desire, but can't be aroused, don't assume it's PD. Have yourself examined for other conditions, those which can reduce or block arousal. These include arterial or venous insufficiency, diabetes, other hormonal diseases, and in men, an enlarged prostate. Stop all unnecessary drugs, including over-the-counter drugs and alcohol. See a urologist or a gynecologist and if necessary, you and your partner should see a psychologist or a sex therapist. If you or your partner are depressed or anxious, one or both of you should be treated.

Impotence

How Common Is Impotence in Parkinson Disease?

Impotence is an under-appreciated problem in PD. Most men with PD and some doctors are unaware that PD can cause impotence. There are 1.2 million PD people and as men are affected more than women, it's estimated that there are 660,000 PD men, and that perhaps 25% are impotent ranging from occasional or partial to habitual failure to get or hold an erection. Most men desire sex and this, coupled with impotence, heightens their frustration, results in abstinence, and deepens their social isolation.

Is It Parkinson or Something Else?

PD usually begins around age 60, a time when some men experience impotence related to vascular disease, diabetes, prostatic enlargement, or depression. Thus impotence may not be attributed to PD. Impotence may be an early symptom of PD, one only appreciated in retrospect. Impotence testing can be extensive or limited based on the setting. Thus, if you're impotent with your partner, but have erections upon awakening, your impotence may be psychological.

How Do I Tell My Doctor I'm Impotent?

Impotence must be acknowledged. Many men are reluctant to admit they are impotent, especially to a female doctor. Or, if they do admit it, do so at the end of the visit as an afterthought. This probably reflects ambiguity and embarrassment. It leaves no time for a frank discussion of a sensitive problem. If impotence is important, it alone should be the subject of the doctor's visit and the partner should attend too. If discussing impotence in the presence of your partner is embarrassing, initially see the doctor alone, but you and your partner should recognize that inability to talk as a couple is part of the problem. Some men become obsessed with impotence; if it is all-encompassing it can turn off even a sympathetic partner. The main ingredients for success in treating impotence are a willingness to seek help, to discuss everything openly, and to respect each other's needs.

Viagra

Although there are many treatments for impotence, Viagra has emerged as the main one. The others include injections, mechanical devices, pumps, and implants. These must be discussed with a urologist.

Viagra, taken by mouth, blocks an enzyme in the erectile tissue of the penis called phosphodiesterase. In doing so, Viagra increases the amount of the naturally occurring chemical nitrous oxide. Nitrous oxide relaxes the erectile tissue of the penis, allowing blood to enter, engorge, and enlarge it. In PD, Viagra is effective in 50% of men, more than 50% of the time.

Viagra peaks in 30 to 120 minutes. That's when erection will peak.

Because Viagra relaxes blood vessels, it may drop your blood pressure if you sit, stand, or your head is above your heart. As some men with PD already drop their pressure in these positions, the combined drop from PD and Viagra when mounting or straddling your partner may cause dizziness or even a black-out. If this is so, it's best for you to be beneath your partner.

If you have serious heart disease, a drop in pressure, coupled with the activity of sexual intercourse, may result in a heart attack, or even death. The risk factor is not Viagra, it's heart disease and sex. I tell men with PD who have serious heart disease and are impotent, and want to try Viagra to consult with their cardiologist. If the cardiologist says you can try Viagra, I recommend the following. Start with the lowest dose of Viagra, 25 mg. Take it one hour before you and your partner have agreed to go to bed. Lie down with your partner, side by side, caress each other, fondle each other, and wait until you're hard — then stop! You've shown that Viagra works, that it didn't drop your blood pressure, or cause a heart attack. The next time you and your partner can complete the act — it'll be just as satisfying, and safer.

Pain in Parkinson Disease

It is said, "Pain and PD don't go together." And when pain appears, it is said to be something else, arthritis, bursitis, a bad back, a frozen shoulder, fibromyalgia, a pinched nerve, a sprained muscle, or nerves. But pain is part of PD, and it has many forms. In Chapter 1 you met Melvin, the state senator whose PD started with shoulder pain, pain his doctors attributed to an old football injury. He was treated with anti-inflammatory drugs, arthritis drugs, acupuncture, exercise, massage, and pain killers to no avail. It wasn't until Melvin was diagnosed with PD and his pain disappeared on Sinemet, that it was attributed, correctly, to PD. In Chapter 5 you will learn about discomfort of Restless Legs, a condition associated with PD, and about the cramping pain of dystonia: neck pain, leg pain, and arm pain.

How common is pain is PD? In my own experience, 50% of people with PD at one time complain of pain, and in perhaps 50% of them, 25% of all people with PD, the pain is related to PD and not something else. The pain is related to PD if it fits a pattern, if it's worse where PD is worse, if it is relieved by PD drugs such as Sinemet plus Comtan, and if there's no other cause.

The Pain of Rigidity

In the beginning, before you're diagnosed with PD, like Melvin you may complain of a dull pain, like a sprain. The pain may be described as aching, gnawing, or nagging. The pain is usually confined to a shoulder, the neck, the back, or a hip. These are either major weight-bearing regions (the back, the hip). Or they're pivots around which multi-directional movements occur: side-to-side, up-and-down, back-and-forth, around-and-around. These pivots are the shoulder, the neck, and to a lesser degree the hip. The elbows and knees are pivots that cause uni-directional movements: back-and-forth (flexion and extension).

This pain is probably related to the rigidity of PD that results in the muscles becoming stiffer, less elastic, harder, and more painful to move. This type of pain magically disappears when Sinemet plus Comtan or a dopamine agonist is started.

The Pain of Dystonia

Before you're diagnosed, you may complain of a pain different from Melvin's. The pain may be described as cramping, sharp, stabbing, or throbbing. It's more intense than Melvin's pain. The pain is usually confined to one or both calves, or forearms, or thighs, or upper arms. This pain is probably related to the dystonia of PD that results in the muscles becoming hard. This pain also magically disappears when Sinemet plus Comtan or a dopamine agonist is started. Dystonia is different from rigidity. Although both make the muscles hard, in rigidity the hardness results from the muscles becoming less elastic, whereas in dystonia it results from the muscles contracting without relaxing. You may not be able to tell or describe the difference, but a neurologist with an EMG (electromyogram — a cardiogram of the muscle) can.

Dystonia of the calves, forearms, thighs, or upper arms may be an early symptom of PD, usually in people below age 40 years. It may appear in PD people who are on Sinemet. Usually it appears as Sinemet "wears off," typically in the early morning when Sinemet levels are low. This is called an "off" dystonia. It's worse on the side more affected by PD. It is treated by adding Comtan or a dopamine agonist to prolong Sinemet's effect. The pain of dystonia can appear as Sinemet peaks, called "on" dystonia. It's harder to treat, requiring re-arranging all your drugs to reduce the highs and lows of Sinemet.

Describe the Pain

Only you feel the pain, only you can describe it. Be as specific as you can. The following is helpful.

Location: Where does it hurt most? The shoulder? The Hip? The Back? Does it stay in one place or does it radiate? If so, where? From the shoulder down the arm? From the back to the hip? Knowing how a pain radiates, is like knowing the road on which a car travels.

Intensity: How bad is it? Describe it on a scale from 0 to 10, where 0 is no pain, and 10 feels like your arm (or leg) was yanked-off, or your skin was ripped off. The pain of PD is usually between 4 and 7. It's never a 10.

Duration: There are two parts.

1. How long have you had the pain? Hours? Days? Weeks? Years?
2. During a typical day, how long does it last? From the time you get up till breakfast? Till lunch? Till dinner? All day?

Associations: Is the pain associated with discoloration, inflammation, redness, swelling, or warmth of the overlying skin? The pain of PD shouldn't be associated with any of the above.

Position: What, if any, positions make it better. What, if any, make it worse.

Quality: There are many ways to describe pain. Some have special meaning. Words used include: aching, biting, burning, cramping (like a charley horse), gripping (like being caught in between a pair of pliers), hurting, nipping, pinching, ripping, smarting, stabbing, and throbbing.

Unusual Pain

Unusual pain may occur in PD and may be related to muscle spasm (from dystonia) with pressure on an underlying nerve. Although it is the muscle that's in spasm, the pain is from the nerve. The pain is more intense than a muscle spasm and radiates along the nerve. The following may occur:

Spasm of the piriformis muscle (in the buttock) with pressure on the sciatic nerve mimicking the pain from a herniated disc.

Spasm of the gastrocnemius muscle (in back of the calf) with pressure on the peroneal nerve or spasm of the tibialis muscle (in front of the calf) with pressure on the tibialis nerve causing calf or foot pain. This may be responsible for the intense leg or foot pain people experience when Sinemet wears off.

Spasm of the pronator muscle in the forearm with pressure on the median nerve or spasm of the extensor muscles of the wrist with pressure on the radial nerve with pain down the forearm.

If spasm of a muscle is the cause of the underlying nerve pain, the treatment is injecting botulinum toxin into the muscle, reducing the spasm and freeing up the nerve.

A diffuse, not well-localized, burning or throbbing pain may sometimes occur in an arm or a leg, or across the chest. Whether this is related to PD, or anxiety, or depression is difficult to pin down. It probably results from a disordered autonomic nervous system.

Treatment

Pain resulting from PD usually responds to PD medication: Sinemet plus Comtan or a dopamine agonist. Pain that responds in part, or pain that's not PD, may be treated as such pain is usually treated. Because many PD people have sensitive stomachs (see *The Stomach in Parkinson Disease,* page 70), I prefer drugs such as Celebrex or Vioxx, drugs that decrease pain but rarely upset the stomach or cause bleeding. Anxiety and depression make pain — the pain from rigidity, dystonia, or a disordered autonomic nervous system — worse. Master your anxiety, and your depression and your pain may disappear.

CHAPTER

5

Parkinson-Like Diseases: Diseases Mistaken for Parkinson

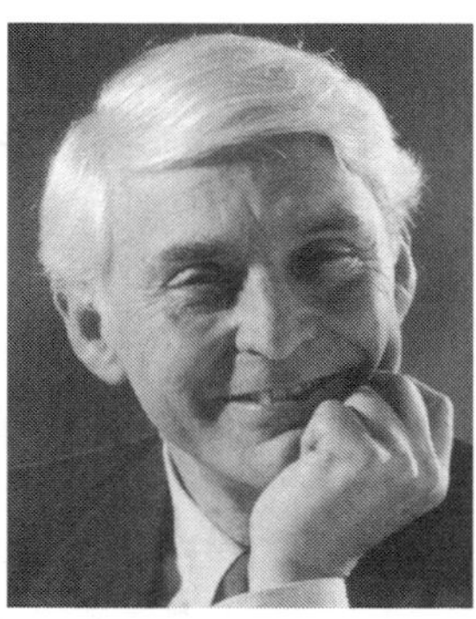

Earl Ubell,
Contributing Editor,
***Parade* magazine**

"When I first learned I had Parkinson disease, I went to see a doctor who told me I was lucky. And I said, 'How do you consider having Parkinson disease lucky?' He told me that if it were any other neurological disease, there would be nothing he could do for me. But today we have drugs, surgery, and a lot of other things like exercise, that will slow things down."

"I've realized how important exercise is to keep your muscles strong. And one hopes that when really good treatments come along, even better than the ones we have now, that you will not have wasted your limbs waiting for them."

"I think I'm better off than other people because I have always exercised. I played tennis. I swam. I used to ride my bike every year in France for two weeks. So between the bicycling, and the tennis, and the trips abroad, I have been keeping in pretty good shape.

"I've had Parkinson disease for nine years. I'm doing well because, number one, I pay attention to what the physician says, and follow the instructions scrupulously. The second most important thing is to continue exercising. You should take every potential possibility for improvement and grab it, because they are few and far between.

"Lately, I've been taking exercise for my speech. I'm really pushing my voice, because I don't want to sound weak. I have taken speech therapy in addition to physical therapy. I think that just keeps me going. I don't get better, but I don't get worse.

"I once asked a clinician, 'How do you explain this? I have practically no trembles, none of the usual things?' And he said, 'You probably started treating it early.'

"At a Board of Directors meeting of one of the organizations with which I work, a very famous doctor was there, and he said, 'How are you doing?' I said, 'I'm doing fine.' And I walked across the floor and tripped on a book and nearly broke my neck. So I guess my timing is still good."

Essential Tremor

Essential tremor (ET) is often mistaken for Parkinson. Essential tremor is more common than PD. For each person with PD there are 10 with ET. Occasionally PD and ET occur together. Although the exact number of people with ET is unknown, it is known that ET increases with age. Although ET occurs in children, the older you are, starting at age 50 years, the more likely you are to develop ET. Although ET is 10 times more common than PD, for every 10 PD people who see a doctor, one ET person sees a doctor. This reflects the benign nature of ET. Whereas PD affects men more than women — 55 men to every 45 women — ET affects men and women equally.

Essential tremor is often called benign essential tremor, because it rarely results in disability. ET is also called familial tremor because in about 50% of people there is a family history. ET is called senile tremor because it is more common among senior citizens. Senile refers to the age at which ET occurs, not to the person's mental capacity. Because of the misleading association of the term senile tremor with senility or mental decline senile tremor isn't used.

Describing Essential Tremor

Essential tremor is characterized by a tremor usually of the hands. The tremor usually begins in both hands unlike the tremor of PD, which begins first in one hand and later the other. ET usually begins insidiously with a person being unaware of it until it is pointed out. ET usually begins in the 2nd, 3rd, 4th, or 5th finger — where it is less likely to be noticed. This is unlike the tremor of PD, which usually begins in the thumb and is more likely to be noticed. The tremor of ET consists of a regular and rhythmical up-and-down movement of each involved finger. The frequency, 5 to 12 beats per minute, is faster than PD. Occasionally the tremor has a circular or rotatory component. Although the tremor usually begins in both hands simultaneously, in about 10% of people the tremor begins in one hand, resulting in confusion with PD.

The tremor of ET reveals itself or increases when people use their hands in an activity such as bringing a glass of water to the lips, tying shoes, or threading a needle. This is called an action or a kinetic tremor. The tremor of ET increases when people stretch out their hands, contracting their muscles to maintain or sustain a fixed position. This is called a postural or sustention tremor. Most ET people have both a postural and an action tremor. In people with ET who have both a postural and an action tremor the postural tremor is usually more obvious. Although 10% of people with PD may have an action or a postural tremor, and 10% of people with ET may have a resting tremor, the other features of the tremor, and the associated finding of PD, such as rigidity and slowness of movement, distinguish PD from ET. All tremors increase with anxiety and disappear during sleep, which makes distinguishing among tremors difficult.

In some ET people the tremor markedly increases when performing a goal-directed action, as in taking the finger and touching the nose. This type of tremor is called an intention tremor. Some ET people have postural, kinetic, and intention tremors with the postural trembling dominating. Some ET people have action and intention tremors. In them the action tremor dominates. Some ET people have only an intention tremor; usually, an isolated intention tremor, one not associated with a postural or action tremor, indicates disease of the cerebellum. The cerebellum is an oval structure about 10% the size of the brain. The cerebellum sits below the brain and behind the brainstem. The name, cerebellum, means "little brain." The cerebellum helps coordinate movement and balance.

Progression of Essential Tremor

The tremor of ET may remain unchanged for years. Or it may change in amplitude and distribution. The changes are slow, but in some people, as time passes, the tremor increases and they develop varying degrees of disability. The disability results solely from the tremor unlike PD where the disability results from the slowness of movement. Eventually, some ET people develop difficulty performing everyday tasks such as holding or handling small objects, tools, or utensils. And some ET people may have difficulty writing, drinking from a cup, feeding themselves, applying makeup, shaving, or dressing.

The tremor in ET may involve the head, the voice, the legs, or trunk. In some people the tremor may start in the head, the voice, or the tongue. A tremor that starts in a hand or a foot on the same side of the body or in the jaw is more likely to be PD. In ET a head, voice, tongue, leg, or trunk tremor may occur in isolation or may be associated with a hand tremor. In ET people the head tremor usually occurs in a horizontal plane and is called a "no-no" tremor; sometimes the head tremor occurs in a vertical plane and is called a "yes-yes" tremor; and sometimes the head tremor occurs in a horizontal and vertical plane and is called a "complex" tremor. In people with an isolated head tremor, the head tremor usually results from dystonia, not ET. This is discussed later in the chapter.

Occasionally in people with ET the voice tremor increases and speech becomes shaky and difficult to understand. This must be distinguished from a spastic dysphonia. Some people with ET, especially those over age 70 years, may become unsteady and have difficulty walking.

Diagnosing Essential Tremor and Distinguishing It from Parkinson

To diagnose a tremor as ET the tremor must be present for at least two years. *All of us, under certain conditions, will tremble — will have a tremor.* Anxiety, fear, uncertainty, worry, and depression can cause all of us to tremble. This tremor, called a physiological tremor, differs from ET in being faster (more beats per second), finer (lower amplitude), and in disappearing when the conditions causing it disappear.

Several conditions including caffeine or nicotine use or withdrawal, alcohol abuse or withdrawal, lithium toxicity, an electrolyte imbalance, a calcium deficiency or excess, and an over-active thyroid can result in a tremor — one that resembles ET. The tremor associated with these conditions disappears when the condition is corrected.

People who develop a tremor are most concerned it is PD. The following characteristics are helpful in distinguishing ET from PD.

1. In ET a postural or action tremor starts in both hands simultaneously. In PD a resting tremor begins in one hand.
2. In ET, after two years, the tremor is not associated with the other symptoms of PD. In PD, after two years, what started as an isolated tremor will now be associated with other symptoms.

3. In ET there may be head tremor. In PD, there may be a tremor confined to the chin or jaw.
4. In ET there is a strong family history. Several members of the same generation may have a tremor. For example, brothers, sisters, and first cousins, and several members of one or more older or younger generations may have a tremor. Or, mothers, fathers, aunts, uncles, grandmothers, grandfathers, grand aunts and uncles, children, nephews, and nieces. In PD, although 15% of people have a family history, it is confined to one or two members of the same generation, or one or two members of an older or younger generation, rarely to several members of the same generation, and rarely to more than two generations.
5. In ET the frequency of the tremor, as measured by an accelerometer, is more rapid (5 to 12 beats per minute) than the tremor of PD (4 to 7 beats per minute).
6. In ET the tremor can be temporarily suppressed by alcohol. In PD the effects of alcohol on suppressing tremor are inconsistent. Alcohol, however, is not a treatment for ET. In time, ever higher amounts of alcohol are needed to suppress the tremor. And, eventually alcohol fails to suppress the tremor. Becoming dependent on alcohol as a treatment for ET can result in the person becoming an alcoholic.
7. In ET, Mysoline, a drug used in epilepsy, can suppress the tremor in some people. Inderal, a drug used in slowing the heart and/or lowering blood pressure may also suppress the tremor as may Remeron, a drug used in depression. And in some people the tremor can be suppressed by Klonopin or Xanax drugs used in treating anxiety. In PD the effects of these drugs on suppressing tremor are inconsistent.

Multiple System Atrophy (MSA)

Among the PD-like diseases is multiple system atrophy in which loss of cells in multiple brain regions, or systems, leads to problems similar to those in PD. However, because the loss of cells is more widespread than in PD, the disability is more severe. Although the drugs for PD may help, success is inconsistent.

The Different Types of Multiple System Atrophy

Because a number of brain regions are affected and because at any one time the effects on one system may overshadow the effects on the others, three types of multiple system atrophy are recognized.

1. When multiple system atrophy starts with difficulty in balance, lack of coordination, and difficulty speaking it is called Olivo-Ponto-Cerebellar Atrophy (OPCA). This indicates the process is affecting the cerebellum and the parts of the brainstem to which it connects: the olives and pons.
2. When multiple system atrophy starts like PD (but without a tremor) and doesn't respond or responds poorly to Sinemet plus Comtan, it is called striato nigral degeneration (SND). This indicates the process affects the same systems as those in PD — but more so.
3. When multiple system atrophy starts with autonomic symptoms (difficulty with urinating, impotence, drop in blood pressure upon standing, fullness of the stomach, loss of sweating or excess sweating, and constipation) it is called Shy Drager after the men who identified it, Milton Shy and Thomas Drager. This indicates that the process affects the autonomic nervous system as well as the systems affected in PD.

Describing Multiple System Atrophy

Multiple system atrophy is uncommon. For every 100 people with PD, there are 2 to 5 people with multiple system atrophy. Multiple system atrophy usually occurs after age 50 and is slightly more common in men than women. Orthostatic hypotension, a drop in blood pressure of 20 millimeters of mercury, results in symptoms upon standing of dizziness, feeling lightheaded, blurred vision, yawning, confusion, and slurred speech. If the drop in blood pressure is marked, the person may faint. Although the blood pressure is low on standing, the blood pressure may be high on lying down. This is called supine hypertension and makes it difficult to regulate blood pressure in a person with multiple system atrophy, trying to steer a course between too high or too low a pressure. Hoarseness is common and vocal paralysis can occur. Such paralysis can be life-threatening, requiring a tracheotomy — the placement of a breathing tube into the throat. Difficulty swallowing is common and, in some people, can result in an inability to swallow, requiring a gastrotomy — the placement of a feeding tube into the stomach.

Distinguishing Multiple System Atrophy from Parkinson

Although, in time, it is apparent who has PD and who has multiple system atrophy, in the beginning the two are confused, even by experts. Multiple system atrophy progresses more quickly than PD, with disability occurring within 5 to 10 years. Although multiple system atrophy may begin as a cerebellar, or a PD-like disease, or an autonomic disease, the diseases may blend.

Recently, an unusual substance has been found in certain types of cells in the brain called glial cells or support cells because they feed and protect the nerve cells. There are about 10 to 100 support cells for each of the 10 billion nerve cells. The support cells in one brain region may be different from those in another. Glial cells contain protein not found in nerve cells. In multiple system atrophy an accumulation of such proteins may lead to the death of the glial cells with secondary death of the nearby nerve cells. The Lewy body, representing an abnormal accumulation of several proteins in nerve cells in PD, is not found in multiple system atrophy. Understanding how proteins accumulate in glial and nerve cells holds the promise to understanding PD and multiple system atrophy and devising ways to prevent or cure both diseases.

Lenny, a 60-Year-Old Man with Shy Drager

I was 50 years old when I became impotent. Laurie, my wife, and I have been married for 30 years. We have three children. I'm a real-estate developer and Laurie and I have been through bankruptcy twice and Hodgkin's disease in Laurie when Hodgkin's was a "death sentence." So impotence wasn't Armageddon.

We saw a urologist who asked many embarrassing questions: "Did Laurie excite me?" She did. "Were we into 'kinky' sex?" We weren't. He checked my prostate: large but not enough to cause impotence. He had me see a vascular man, an endocrinologist, and a neurologist — none of whom could explain my impotence. Then he had Laurie and I see a sex therapist in case we'd been too embarrassed to tell the urologist everything. The therapist was baffled: the impotence was physical not psychological. But she didn't know why. She recommended Laurie inject a hormone: prostaglandin into my penis before we had sex. Prostaglandin brings blood into the penis and keeps it there. The injections didn't work. Neither would Viagra — were it available.

Next, I developed difficulty urinating: frequency, hesitancy, and urgency. Each night I'd get up frequently to urinate. And each day I'd frequently get the urge to urinate, I'd hesitate — and nothing would happen. I returned to my urologist who said it was my prostate. So he removed it — but the symptoms continued. I'm glad the impotence came before I had the surgery — or else I would've blamed the surgery and been guilt-stricken for going through with it.

I tried several drugs to control the urination. The best was Detrol. It helped but then I became constipated. My urologist was certain it was Detrol so I stopped it — but the constipation continued. Then my bladder stopped working — I couldn't pee! I re-started the Detrol but it no longer helped and Laurie had to learn to catheterize me. For the constipation I saw a gastroenterologist. She examined every inch of my gut — and came up with nothing. She recommended fiber: at least 20 grams a day. And stool softeners. And exercise to build up my abdominal muscles: to help in pushing out my stool. And they helped.

Then I became wobbly. Part of it was dizziness when I stood up. And part of it was unsteadiness: my legs would sway and wouldn't hold me. I felt as though I was drunk but I wasn't. Laurie noticed it and I returned to the neurologist. He asked me many questions and put me through a long and detailed examination. "The dizziness," he said, "results from your blood pressure dropping when you stand up. The drop in blood pressure, the unsteadiness, the bladder difficulty, the constipation, and the impotence are related. I think I know how — but I need more data."

He ordered an MRI of the brain, the upper, the middle, and the lower spinal cord: every inch of my nervous system — and all normal. "I thought they'd be normal — but I had to be sure. You have Shy Drager," he said.

"What is Shy Drager?" Laurie asked. "And is it curable?"

"It is a Parkinson-like disease also called multiple system atrophy," he replied. "In addition to affecting the same parts of the brain as Parkinson, it affects the autonomic nervous system, the part that regulates blood pressure, bowel, bladder, and sexual function. The autonomic nervous system is affected by Parkinson but not as severely and or as early as in Shy Drager. It is not curable — and there are few treatments."

When Laurie had Hodgkin's disease I could see the tumor. But Shy Drager was like "boxing with shadows." Laurie and I had faced difficult times: Hodgkin's disease, bankruptcy. While we couldn't see Shy Drager at least we had a name. And "boxing with Shy Drager" was better than "boxing with a shadow."

I won't tell you the next few years were a "Garden of Eden." I manage the dizziness on standing by drinking a balanced salt solution: Gatorade. It keeps my circulation full and prevents my blood pressure from dropping. Sort of "dehydration" in reverse. And I take Proamatine which restores, in part, the tone of my blood vessels. I should wear thigh length elastic stockings but they're hard to put on, hard to pull off — and not for me.

Recently I developed difficulty swallowing. The Parkinson (or Shy Drager) process involves the muscles of swallowing including the tongue which pushes food into the throat, the throat muscles which "massage" the food into the gullet, and the gullet muscles which "massage" the food into the stomach. The throat muscles also close off the wind-pipe, stopping food from getting into my lungs. But sometimes my muscles "fall down on the job" — and I gag. Although the muscles of swallowing and speaking are the same, and I was told my speaking would be affected — it hasn't. I went to a speech therapist who taught me how the muscles of speech and swallowing work, how to strengthen them — and what steps I could take to lead a normal life. I practice her instructions daily — and they help.

A physical therapist taught me that riding a reclining bicycle, walking in a warm pool, and massage help: my muscles are toned and my feet don't swell. Going out is a chore, so Laurie and I entertain at home: we have people over at least twice a week. Sinemet and Comtan, which aren't supposed to help Shy Drager — help. They help my swallowing, my writing, and my turning in bed. And they help, in part, my unsteadiness: my legs feel stronger after I take them. My neurologist is skeptical but when I cut back I have more difficulty swallowing, writing, turning in bed, and walking. My neurologist doesn't know my body and brain as well as I do.

Laurie and I became close after she was diagnosed with Hodgkin's disease. I was her counselor, her care partner and now she's mine. And neither of us have regrets about taking care of the other. We're active in our Parkinson support group — Laurie's the president. Shy Drager is uncommon: for every 100 people with Parkinson there are 2 to 5 with Shy Drager. So there aren't many Shy Drager support groups. The group meets in our home and my office helps with the newsletter and events. Helping others and giving of yourself is a powerful treatment: better than Detrol, Gatorade, and Sinemet.

Recently I took the Quality of Life Exam and did as follows:

My Mobility Index is 33 (out of 40 points).

My Emotional Index is 7 (out of 44 points).

My Autonomic Index is 13 (out of 16 points).

My Total Score on the Quality of Life Scale is 53%.

Despite my difficulty with mobility and body functions I consider my Quality of Life to be good.

If you didn't know, we read the Bible every day. I quote from the Book of Psalms.

GOD, DO NOT REBUKE ME IN ANGER, NOR PUNISH ME IN WRATH.
HEAL ME BECAUSE I TREMBLE, AND MY SPIRIT IS SHAKEN TO ITS DEPTHS.

I AM WORN DOWN WITH GROANING,
EVERY NIGHT I DRENCH MY PILLOW, AND SOAK MY BED WITH TEARS.
MY EYES WASTE AWAY WITH VEXATION.
BUT GOD WILL HEAR THE SOUND OF MY WEEPING,
AND GOD WILL ACCEPT MY PRAYER.

Progressive Supranuclear Palsy

Progressive supranuclear palsy (PSP) was diagnosed in actor-comedian Dudley Moore, calling attention to a little known disease. Progressive supranuclear palsy is characterized by slow movement (like PD), rigidity (like PD), and postural instability with falls (more striking than PD). Tremor is usually absent (unlike PD). Progressive supranuclear palsy is uncommon. For every 100 people with PD there are 2 to 5 with PSP; 20,000 to 50,000 PSP people versus 1,000,000 PD people in the United States.

Describing Progressive Supranuclear Palsy

Initially, PSP may be mistaken for PD even by experts. In time, the differences become apparent. Progressive supranuclear palsy usually begins about age 60 (like PD), but it progresses more quickly with people becoming disabled within 5 to 10 years.

Often, PSP patients begin with balance difficulty and falls. This is unlike PD, where falls occur later. In PSP rigidity is prominent in the muscles of the neck and spine. Rigidity is less prominent in the arms and legs. And rigidity, when present in the arms and legs, is equal on both sides. This is different from PD. In PSP, the muscles in the back of the neck are usually more affected by rigidity than the muscles in the front of the neck. Consequently, the neck may bend backward — the person looks up at the ceiling. This is called retro-collis. In some PSP people the muscles in the front of the neck are more affected than the muscles in the back of the neck. Consequently, the neck may bend forward — the person looks down at the floor. This is called antero-collis. In PSP the rigidity of the spine can be striking, resulting in a stiff, extended spine. This is unlike the bent, flexed spine of PD.

The Eyes in Progressive Supranuclear Palsy

The most striking symptom in PSP, the symptom for which PSP is named — is eye-movement paralysis. The paralysis occurs early, allowing PSP to be distinguished from PD. In some PSP people, however, eye-movement paralysis occurs late, making it hard to distinguish PSP from PD. Rarely, PSP people have normal eye movements. In these instances the diagnosis has been made at autopsy. Although PD people have eye-movement difficulties, it is rare for PD people to have eye movements as impaired as those with PSP.

In PSP the eyelids may be held wide open. This, coupled with the eye-movement paralysis, results in a facial expression that's described as astonished, puzzled, or staring. It is unlike the grim-masked face of PD. Sometimes in PSP the eyelids shut tightly and cannot be opened. This is called blepharospasm, which is discussed later.

Usually in PSP the patient's eye-movement difficulties begin with looking up or down. Later, the person may have difficulty looking to the right or left. The eye-movement difficulties may impair driving and reading. In PSP the eye muscles are normal. The nerve fibers that carry impulses to the eyes are normal. And the nerve cells located in centers or nuclei that generate the impulses carried by the nerve fibers are normal. These nuclei are in the brainstem near the substantia nigra, the target in PD. Similar but not identical brain regions are targeted in PD and PSP, explaining the similarities between them.

Eye-movement centers above (superior to, or *supra* to) the brainstem where eye-movement nuclei are targeted and paralyzed — hence the name: progressive supranuclear palsy, PSP. Areas near these centers are also targeted and impaired. These areas are in the brainstem.

Progressive Supranuclear Palsy, Parkinson, and the Brainstem

The brainstem consists of three parts:

1. The upper one-third, called the midbrain, which contains the substantia nigra and the eye-movement nuclei. The midbrain is targeted in PD and PSP.

2. The middle one-third, called the pons. Within the pons, fibers from the cerebellum (a balancing center) and fibers controlling leg movement criss-cross and comingle. The pons is targeted in PSP, explaining, perhaps, the early difficulty with balance. The pons is usually not targeted in PD.
3. The lower one-third is called the medulla or "bulb" because of its resemblance to a tulip bulb. The medulla contains nerve cells that control speech and swallowing. Paralysis of the bulb or bulbar palsy results in difficulty speaking and swallowing. The bulb is spared in PSP. However, nerve cells and nerve fibers originating above the bulb, anywhere from the basal ganglia to the pons, are targeted in PSP. This can result in paralysis of speech and swallowing similar to a bulbar palsy. However, as the bulb is normal, the paralysis is called pseudobulbar palsy. Pseudobulbar palsy may be an early or late symptom of PSP. The harsh, grating speech of some PSP people can usually be distinguished from the subdued speech of PD people.

People who suffer from pseudobulbar palsy may also display emotional lability or emotional incontinence. Such people cry easily — often when there's no reason to cry.

Less commonly a person with a pseudobulbar palsy may laugh inappropriately. In pseudobulbar palsy there is a disconnect between the reasons for crying (or laughing) and the facial expression of sadness (or joy) and production of tears (or laughter). Thus a bland or innocent remark will trigger crying (or laughing) even when the person is not sad (or happy). Pseudobulbar palsy occurs in other disorders which damage the brainstem, such as multiple strokes or head injuries.

Other, less common PSP symptoms include gasps during inspiration, grunts during expiration, peculiar breathing, and muscle jerks. In PSP, standard laboratory tests are normal (as in PD). The diagnosis is made from the person's history and the peculiarities on examination — especially the eye movements. Late in PSP, usually after the diagnosis is made, the MRI may show atrophy (shrinkage) of the brainstem (unlike in PD). Occasionally, the brainstem atrophy is present early in PSP, easing the diagnosis. PSP people respond minimally, temporarily, or not at all to PD drugs. Indeed, if a person is diagnosed with PD and shows little response to Sinemet plus Comtan, a PD-like disease is suspected.

What Causes Progressive Supranuclear Palsy?

Post-mortem examination of the PSP brain reveals distinctive features. There is atrophy (varying from moderate to marked) of the brainstem. Less marked is atrophy of the cerebellum. The brainstem and cerebellum show gliosis, a type of scarring in which normal tissue nerve cells are replaced by glial cells. The glial cells and the nerve cells arise from a primitive cell called the stem cell. As nerve cells die they may be replaced by glial cells, forming a scar. The glial cells are unable to duplicate the function of the nerve cells. Some of the dying nerve cells contain spaces partly filled with fine particles or granules. This type of change also occurs in the cortex of people with Alzheimer disease.

Most of the dying nerve cells contain twisted, tangled fibers made up of a partially crystallized protein, the tau protein. This type of change commonly occurs in the cortex of people with Alzheimer disease. Amyloid plaques are made up of deposits of a protein called amyloid outside the dying cells, another feature of Alzheimer disease that occurs in PSP. In general, so similar are the changes in the brainstem of PSP people with the changes in the brains of Alzheimer people that PSP has been called "Alzheimer of the brainstem." While Alzheimer and PSP are alike, the mind is spared in PSP.

Changes similar to PSP, as well as changes in the brain and spinal cord, occur in the Parkinson Disease Dementia — amyotrophic lateral sclerosis (Lou Gehrig's disease) of Guam. This disease affects up to 10% of the natives of Guam. Some have symptoms of PD and Alzheimer disease, some have symptoms of Lou Gehrig's disease, some have symptoms of PSP and some have symptoms of all. Understanding how proteins accumulate in cells holds the promise of understanding and eventually curing all of these diseases.

Eye Problems in Parkinson Disease

A discussion of PSP leads to a discussion of a little-emphasized problem in PD: the eyes and sight. Difficulty seeing includes difficulty reading, visual blurring, difficulty keeping the eyes open, and hallucinations. Hallucinations, seeing objects or people no one else sees, is discussed later. Many eye problems are related to aging, not PD. A PD person with difficulty seeing should first consult an eye doctor to be certain the difficulty isn't related to glaucoma, cataracts, or macular degeneration.

Eye Problems and Parkinson Drugs

Certain Parkinson drugs, the anticholinergic drugs, such as Artane, Akineton, and Cogentin; certain drugs for depression, such as the tricyclic drugs that have anticholinergic properties; and certain drugs used to treat overactive bladders that have anticholinergic properties can increase eye pressure, especially in people with a type of glaucoma called narrow-angle glaucoma. If you have PD and glaucoma and are taking an anticholinergic drug you should check with your eye doctor.

The Eyelids

Early in PD, before treatment, the lids and the muscles controlling them become rigid. This results in retraction of the lids, causing the person to stare or look startled. This is more marked in PSP. In addition, in PD the frequency of blinking is decreased. This is an early symptom of PD. Sometimes the lids go into spasm, closing forcibly and staying closed for hours, a condition called blepharospasm. Blepharospasm is a form of dystonia. Blepharospasm can be improved, worsened, or unaffected by PD drugs. Blepharospasm is treated by injections of botulinum toxin, a drug that weakens the lids, stopping them from closing involuntarily while allowing them to close voluntarily.

Some PD people tear and seem to be crying. Tearing may result from rigidity of the lower lid. The lower lid acts as a cup to catch, hold, and re-circulate tears that are normally formed and lubricate the eyes. If the lid is rigid, it no longer acts like a cup, and instead of being retained, tears flow down the cheeks. Often, as the rigidity lessens, the lower lids again form a "cup" and the tearing stops. Dry eyes, the opposite of tearing, may result from underactivity of the parasympathetic nervous system.

The Pupils

The pupils or camera shutters are unaffected in PD. However, some of the drugs used in treating PD, the anticholinergic drugs, dilate or widen the pupil, causing blurring. The blurring may be pronounced when you read. If we compare the eye to a camera, the smaller the opening of the camera, the sharper the image on the retina. The wider the opening of the eye the fuzzier the image.

The Eye Muscles

There are six eye muscles in each eye. Two muscles move the eyeball from side-to-side. One muscle is controlled by a nerve, Cranial Nerve 6, that starts in the brainstem. The other muscle is controlled by a nerve, Cranial Nerve 3, that also starts in the brainstem near the substantia nigra, where PD starts. Two muscles move the eyeball up and down. These muscles are controlled by Cranial Nerve 3. Cranial Nerve 3 also carries the fibers that narrow the pupil. Two muscles rotate the eye ball. One is controlled by a nerve, Cranial Nerve 4, that starts in a part of the brainstem near where PD starts. Given the origin of two of the Cranial Nerves, numbers 3 and 4, near where PD starts, it's surprising, happily, that problems seeing aren't more frequent in PD.

The eye muscles aren't affected, as far as we can tell, by the rigidity and slowness of movement that affect other muscles in PD.

Nonetheless, it's possible that some of the difficulty "seeing," especially in reading, may result from subtle difficulties in the muscles. A common difficulty, convergence insufficiency, in which both eyes must simultaneously approach each other — as in holding an object (such as a book) up close and reading it — may result, in part, from such a difficulty. Some of these problems can be corrected by prisms.

Eye Movements and the Brainstem

Eye movements have fast and slow components that are studied with an Electro Nystagmogram (ENG). Three types of eye movements, detected on the ENG, may be relevant to PD.

1. The "fast movement" brings images in the periphery to bear on the fovea, the sensitive part of the retina. Normally such a fast movement brings the image from the periphery into focus on the fovea in a single move. In PD, the time from when the image is seen to when the fast movement starts, is delayed. This is the eye movement equivalent of bradykinesia. Usually if you anticipate seeing an image, you start the fast movement. Often, the person with PD, when anticipating seeing an image, can't start the fast movement. This is the eye movement equivalent of freezing. As PD progresses, eye-movement bradykinesia and eye-movement freezing become more pronounced. These delays in movement cannot be appreciated without an ENG. They may be partly responsible for the difficulty seeing in PD, a difficulty that cannot be appreciated during a routine examination.
2. *The low amplitude, smooth pursuit movement.* This movement tracks a predictably moving target, such as a plane traveling at a given speed, or a golf ball traveling at a given speed. The low amplitude smooth pursuit movement is slowed in PD and may

explain why some PD people complain of difficulty following moving objects.

3. *The scanning eye movement* is used in looking through a field of objects while searching for a specific object. This scanning may be slowed in PD, resulting in an ability to distinguish among objects of similar colors, shapes, or sizes. This could result in blurred vision.

Restless Legs

Restless legs is not a PD-like disease, however, it occurs in people with and without PD. The prevalence of restless legs isn't known, but is estimated at 1% or 2.8 million Americans. About 5% of people with restless legs seek treatment. Some doctors argue restless legs is a predicator of PD. Restless legs is characterized by unpleasant leg sensations. The sensations occur at night during sleep when the leg muscles are relaxed. The sensations result in an irresistible desire to move the legs to the point of getting up and walking. Restless legs usually occurs early in the morning, waking people from sleep.

The legs appear normal. But studies in sleep laboratories show leg movements throughout the night in 80% of people with restless legs. The movements consist of extension of the big toe and foot and flexion of the knee.

Restless legs occurs in PD people before and during treatment. Rarely, restless legs may be the first symptom of PD. Treatment for restless legs includes benzodiazepines: Klonopin, Restoril, and Valium. Benzodiazepines improve the nighttime sleep but don't affect the leg movements. Benzodiazepines are addictive, cause daytime drowsiness, and are discouraged as initial therapy for restless legs. Long-acting Sinemet-CR plus Comtan, or a dopamine agonist such as Mirapex taken at bedtime reduces restless legs in people with and without PD. This may be related to a decrease in dopamine in the spinal cord, which may be the basis of restless legs.

Dystonia

Dystonia is a symptom of PD affecting multiple muscles and restricted muscle groups. Rarely, some forms of dystonia in children may be mistaken for PD.

Describing Dystonia

Dystonia is characterized by contractions of muscles resulting in painful, twisting-turning movements and aberrant postures. Dystonia is classified into primary dystonia (dystonia without a cause) and secondary dystonia (dystonia that occurs after a stroke or with PD). Dystonia in children usually starts in one leg, spreads to the trunk, then the arms, and then the neck. It is often familial. Dystonia in adults is usually restricted to one or more limbs, the neck, or muscles of the face. Dystonia in adults starts in the thirties to fifties (earlier than PD), and affects three women for every man. For every five people with PD there's one with dystonia.

Dystonia's onset is gradual with symptoms varying depending on the muscles affected and their degree of spasm. Dystonia progresses initially then stabilizes. Symptoms can be intermittent, appearing during times of stress, then disappearing. The most common types of dystonia are described below.

1. **Blepharospasm.** People with blepharospasm can have intermittent or sustained eyelid closure as a result of contraction of the eyelid muscles. Blepharospasm occurs in people with or without PD. It is more common in people without PD. When the spasms are limited to the lids the disorder is called essential blepharospasm. Blepharospasm may begin in one eye — but soon involve the other. Initially, symptoms consist of excessive blinking, irritation, and burning of the eyes, and photophobia. People with blepharospasm may have difficulty reading, watching television, or driving. Blepharospasm is aggravated by stress, looking up or down, reading,

driving, and bright light. For this reason people with blepharospasm wear dark glasses.

Tricks that temporarily relieve blepharospasm include talking, lying down, singing, yawning, laughing, chewing, and eyebrow pressure. The best treatment is injections of botulinum toxin into the muscles of the eyelids.

2. **Spasmodic Dysphonia.** Spasmodic dysphonia, resulting from spasm of the vocal cords, was originally described as a form of hysterical hoarseness and was wrongly considered to be psychogenic. Vocal cord spasm occurs during speech and disappears during silence. Spasmodic dysphonia occurs in people with and without PD. It is more common in people without PD. There are two types of cord spasm. In one, the cords come together, they adduct. In the second, the cords move apart, they abduct. This is caused by spasm of the surrounding muscles (especially the posterior cricoarytenoid muscles). People with adductor spasm speak in a choked, strained, or strangled voice. The speech is characterized by frequent breaks. Abductor spasm is less frequent. People with abductor spasm speak in a breathy, whispering voice. Distinguishing adductor from abductor spasm requires seeing the vocal cords through a laryngoscope.

   Tricks that help, temporarily, are yawning or sneezing. The best treatment is injections of botulinum toxin into the vocal cords.

3. **Wry Neck or Spasmodic Torticollis** (ST). Dystonia of the neck muscles results in a wry or twisted neck. Spasmodic torticollis is the most common dystonia: it is five times more common than all the other dystonias combined. People with spasmodic torticollis start with jerky movements of the head, followed by twisting of the face to one side or the other, or, less

commonly, twisting of the neck backward (retro collis) or forward (antero collis). Often the shoulder is elevated on the side toward which the face turns. A charley horse type of pain is frequent. A head tremor resulting from spasm of opposing neck muscles occurs in 30% of people. Spasmodic torticollis does not occur in PD except as a complication of Sinemet treatment.

The best treatment is injections of botulinum toxin into the dystonic muscles.

4. **Writer's Cramp.** Writer's cramp results from a dystonic spasm of the muscle that extends the thumb. Writer's cramp may start as a tremor of the hand. The tremor is usually present in one position, the position which stretches the muscles that extend the thumb. Writer's cramp appears as an inability to write legibly while other actions of the thumb are normal.

   The best treatment is injections of botulinum toxin into the dystonic muscles.

People ask, if God created the world, and if God is good, why did God create Parkinson Disease, progressive supranuclear palsy, multiple system atrophy, and dystonia? Read Isaiah; God has a purpose, we may not understand it.

Isaiah
Did you not know? Have you not heard?
People grow tired and weary,
They stumble and fall.
But those who believe in God regain their strength.
They sprout wings like eagles.
And though they run they do not grow weary
And though they walk they do not tire.

CHAPTER

6

The Causes of Parkinson Disease

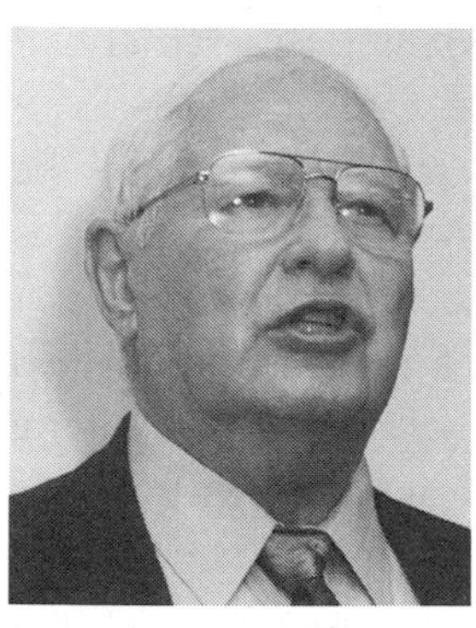

Jack Anderson, Columnist

"I was diagnosed with Parkinson disease about a dozen years ago. First, it was just a twitch of the right thumb, and I thought, 'Uh-oh, old age is catching up with me.' Then, a couple of fingers began to twitch, and then the whole hand. And at that, I got alarmed. So I went to see the doctor, and the doctor said it was Parkinson. I was not happy at the news. My brother also has Parkinson and so I had a preview. He would tell me what was happening to him and I knew that soon it would happen to me. I've always known exactly where I'm headed, what curses are going to come upon me and I've just had to put up with it.

"I reserve one hour a day to feel sorry for myself. It's from seven to eight in the morning. At eight o'clock, I end all that. I have no more time to feel sorry for myself; I've got too many things to do. And I go out and do them.

"I believe that this problem is solvable. The researchers now working on it are the most zealous, committed people I've ever met. We haven't solved it yet, but we can, and we will."

In 95% of people with PD the cause is unknown — hence the name *idiopathic PD*. In under 5% a cause is known. Among the known causes are viruses, brain injuries, heavy metals, chemicals, and genetics. In this chapter some of these causes are discussed.

Did A Virus Cause Adolf Hitler's Parkinson Disease?

Adolf Hitler had PD. This fact surprises most people because Hitler, the most evil man of the 20th century, was also the most photographed. And when PD appears, it is easily recognized. So how could the German public not know Hitler had PD? How could the Allies, England, Russia, and the United States, possessors of sophisticated secret services using thousands of spies, not know Hitler had PD? If an American President had PD, would we know?

In 1940 Hitler developed a tremor in his left hand. After this, he was rarely seen. He limited his public appearances and let himself be filmed only from angles that did not show his tremor. But he may not have realized he had PD. By 1945 his PD was advanced. A Swedish newsreel of the time shows Hitler walking slowly and not swinging his left arm. He has a masked, dull, expressionless face. He is stooped and bent forward, and has a marked tremor of his left arm. Hitler's earliest symptom, decreased movement of his left arm, is seen in Leni Reifenstahl's 1934 film, *Triumph of the Will.* Hitler, like most people with PD, was unaware his left arm was not moving.

Eyewitness reports attesting to Hitler's PD include:

- General Guderian, Hitler's Chief of Staff, writing in 1943: "Hitler's left hand trembled, his back was bent, and his gaze was fixed."

- Albert Speer, Hitler's architect, writing in 1944: "Hitler was shriveling up like an old man. His limbs trembled, he walked stooped with dragging footsteps. His uniform, which in the past he'd kept clean, was stained by the food he'd eaten with his shaking hands."
- General von Cholitz, Hitler's Commander in Paris, saying upon meeting Hitler in 1944: "He had become an old man. His face was worn. His shoulders sagged. He cupped his left hand in his right to hide the trembling of his left arm. But it was his voice that shocked me. The hard raucous voice had faded to a weak whisper."
- Hitler had micrographia, the cramped handwriting characteristic of PD.

In 1918 Hitler was taken to a military hospital after being gassed. There he may have caught encephalitis. An epidemic of encephalitis lethargica, "sleeping sickness," swept the world from 1918 to 1926, infecting more than 15 million people, 6 million of whom developed PD. Many developed PD immediately. For some patients their symptoms were permanent, while in others symptoms disappeared only to reappear years later; many who had never had PD initially developed it years later. The time from infection until the appearance of PD varied from 1 to 25 years. This disease was called post-encephalitis Parkinson to distinguish it from idiopathic PD. The symptoms of post-encephalitis Parkinson were similar to those of idiopathic PD. The diseases differed at post-mortem examination. In post-encephalitis Parkinson, as in idiopathic PD, there was a loss of cells in the substantia nigra but, unlike in idiopathic PD, there were no Lewy bodies. The post-mortem changes in post-encephalitis Parkinson resembled the changes in progressive supranuclear palsy (PSP).

Unless a person had a history of encephalitis, it was difficult to tell these diseases apart — short of a post-mortem examination. Hitler was in a hospital, there was an epidemic of encephalitis, and people in the hospital had encephalitis. But it is not known for certain if Hitler had encephalitis: his medical records are missing.

During the 1930s and 1940s the number of people with post-encephalitis Parkinson equaled the number with idiopathic PD. As the survivors of the epidemic died off, post-encephalitis Parkinson became more and more uncommon. With the exception of isolated cases from encephalitis caused by agents other than the one that caused the epidemic of 1918 to 1926, there are few people with post-encephalitis Parkinson. Although we do not know for certain that Hitler had encephalitis, there are indications he had post-encephalitis Parkinson.

In the 1930s and 1940s, people with post-encephalitis Parkinson were younger than people with idiopathic PD. In 1934, when Hitler developed PD, he was 45 years old. At that time, a 45-year-old man with PD was more likely to have post-encephalitis Parkinson than idiopathic PD. People with post-encephalitis Parkinson were more likely to have peculiar sleep patterns. Hitler had peculiar sleep patterns: he rarely went to bed before 4 A.M. and rarely woke before noon. Finally, and most characteristically, people with post-encephalitis Parkinson had a peculiar spasm of the eyes, called an oculogyric crisis, a spasm not seen in any other condition. Such a spasm was described in Hitler by several people. The following was reported from an observer at the Munich Conference in 1938: "Suddenly Hitler's face becomes expressionless as he struggles against a spasm of his eyes. He twitches his eyebrows and tilts his head backward as though trying to break the spasm."

Viruses cause encephalitis and can alter the brain. Some can seek out the dopamine cells of the substantia nigra, and, like idiopathic PD, destroy these cells, resulting in post-encephalitis Parkinson. This is what happened to 6 million people between 1918 and 1926, including Adolf Hitler. In idiopathic PD, the process that destroys the dopamine-making cells leaves a calling card — the Lewy body. In post-encephalitis Parkinson, the virus doesn't leave a calling card.

Does Boxing Cause Parkinson?

The following was adapted from an article written by Dr. Ira Casson for the *NPF Parkinson Report*. Dr. Casson is a neurologist and an expert on boxing and the brain.

1. A small number of people, less than 1%, who sustain significant head injuries develop PD or a PD-like disease. Significant head injury means the person was in a coma for 24 hours or more, may have needed surgery to remove a blood clot, and spent several weeks or months in a hospital.
2. Minor head injury does not cause PD. There are people who develop PD who are certain the disease began after a minor head injury. For PD to begin, approximately 60% of the cells in the substantia nigra must be lost. These cells are not lost because of a minor injury. If PD develops after a minor injury, it is likely PD was present and the injury brought it out. A minor head injury is one that does not result in a loss of consciousness. Or, if it does, then the loss of consciousness is brief. Such people are rarely hospitalized.
3. A problem arises when there is a lawsuit and a person claims a blow to his head caused his PD. The scientific evidence does not support this, but how a judge and jury decide may be different.
4. Lastly is the role of boxing. There has been interest in this because of Muhammad Ali. The following can be said: It is uncertain if there is a relationship between Ali's Parkinson and boxing. When boxing causes brain damage, the result is an Alzheimer-like disease. This is not what Ali has; Ali's mind is sharp. It is rare for a boxing injury to result in only PD. And most boxers do not develop Alzheimer or Parkinson. George Foreman is on television doing a fine job selling his grill, and his boxing career lasted longer and he took more blows than Ali.

Boxing and the Brain

Terms such as *dementia pugilistica, chronic encephalopathy,* and *chronic brain injury* have been brought to everyone's attention and created renewed interest in the effects of boxing on the brain. These terms encompass a wide range of disorders. At one end are boxers with minimal damage and at the other end are severely affected boxers requiring institutional care. Within this range are boxers with varying degrees of speech difficulty, stiffness, unsteadiness, memory loss, and inappropriate behavior. There are also a few who are severely affected and give rise to the phrase "punch drunk."

In different studies, 15 – 40% of ex-boxers are found to have symptoms of a brain injury. Most have mild symptoms. Recent studies using detailed psychological testing and MRI scanning have shown that many professional boxers, including those without obvious symptoms, have some degree of brain injury. Although there are still some "punch drunk" fighters, there are fewer today. Today's boxers have fewer fights and shorter careers, resulting in fewer blows to the head and less injury.

Onset of Symptoms

Symptoms usually begin near or shortly after the end of a boxer's career. On occasion they are first noticed after a particularly hard fight. Symptoms develop an average of 16 years after starting to box, although in some symptoms appear as early as six years after starting to box. Symptoms have been reported in boxers as young as 25 years of age. Although brain damage has been reported in amateurs, it is more common in professionals. It can occur in all weight classes but is more common among heavyweights. Champions run a higher risk of chronic injury than journeymen. The evidence suggests that the chronic encephalopathy of boxers is a progressive disorder. The literature contains many case reports of a PD-like disorder that is progressive, even after the boxer has retired.

As the damage accumulates, minimal symptoms merge gradually into more obvious symptoms. The boxer usually is not aware of his difficulties; his wife is often the first to notice subtle personality changes. Extreme intolerance of alcoholic beverages is a common symptom in the early stages. Confrontations with law enforcement authorities are often the result of lost social inhibitions or sudden changes in mood and behavior. The confrontations are often preceded by delusions, violent rages, and morbid jealousy, including repeated accusations of infidelity of the boxer's spouse. These difficulties usually are explained away as symptoms of depression, anxiety, or even the enthusiasm of an immature, aging athlete.

Difficulty with mobility is usually noticed first by the trainer. A lack of coordination, a loss of balance, or a generalized slowing down initially is attributed to the normal aging process. However, as these symptoms worsen, it becomes apparent to the boxer's companions that something is wrong, even though the boxer continues to insist that he is healthy.

Four Types of Disorders Related to Boxing

1. A disorder similar to general paresis (syphilis of the brain) but without syphilis
2. A disorder similar to multiple sclerosis
3. A disorder similar to Alzheimer disease
4. A disorder similar to Parkinson disease

In 1969, in a British study of 224 former boxers, 37 (16%) had evidence of brain damage that could be attributed to boxing and 13 (6%) were severely affected. Speech difficulty is characteristic of all these disorders and is usually present in all brain damage cases. There is a relationship between the length of the boxer's career, the number of bouts, and the prevalence of brain injury. Of those who fought for 10 years, 47% were affected, compared with 13% of those who fought for less than five years. Half of the group who had more than 150 professional bouts showed symptoms of brain damage compared with 19% of those with 50 to 150 professional bouts, and 7% of those who fought fewer than 50 times.

Post-mortem examination of four boxers with a PD-like disorder revealed a loss of dopamine cells in the substantia nigra but without Lewy bodies. This pattern is similar to that seen in post-encephalitis Parkinson.

Boxing can injure the brain. In some boxers the injury includes damage to the substantia nigra, and like idiopathic PD, these destroyed cells result in Parkinson. The way that multiple and repeated blows to the head cause Parkinson is not known, but it appears that the deep areas of the brain including the substantia nigra are most affected by repeated blows. One can argue that every blow to the head results in microscopic damage to the substantia nigra. As the blows continue, this damage increases.

Parkinson Caused by Drugs — Temporary Parkinson

Some drugs cause a PD-like disorder. Unlike PD, which starts, insidiously, on one side and slowly spreads to the other, drug-related Parkinson starts on both sides — simultaneously and often abruptly. In some people, symptoms start after a few days. Usually, however, symptoms start within one to three months. After stopping the drug, symptoms disappear in most people within a few weeks. However, in some people symptoms may last for months. The potentially long duration of symptoms is important to understand in order to avoid diagnosing idiopathic PD. Drug-related symptoms usually improve after stopping the drug, whereas the symptoms of idiopathic PD worsen. The responsible drugs are those that block a receptor in the brain, the D-2 dopamine receptor. Blocking this receptor prevents dopamine from attaching itself to the receptor, resulting in a PD-like disorder. Such drugs called "neuroleptics" are used in psychiatry to treat schizophrenia and other aberrant behaviors. An exception is Reglan, a drug used to treat certain stomach disorders. The problem occurs when after stopping the drug the symptoms remain. This probably means the drug has unmasked a latent PD — a disease that would have appeared even if the drug had not been used. Post-mortem examination of the brains of people who developed drug-related PD are normal; there is no loss of cells in the substantia nigra.

Neuroleptics introduced in the 1950s and 1960s, drugs such as Thorazine, Stellazine, and Haldol, are more likely to cause PD symptoms than current drugs. Indeed Clozaril, an "atypical" neuroleptic, does not cause PD or other symptoms such as dyskinesia, dystonia, restlessness, tremors, or tics. In the 1950s and 1960s the incidence of neuroleptic PD was as high as 25% of all people treated with neuroleptics. Unlike most drug-related side effects, there is no relationship between the drug dose, the duration of treatment, and PD. Side effects of the neuroleptics are not limited to PD.

Anticholinergic drugs are frequently used to treat drug-related PD because they decrease symptoms better than Sinemet or the dopamine agonists. This may be due to the fact that since the dopamine receptor is blocked by the neuroleptic, the dopamine that is generated by Sinemet is not as effective as the anticholinergic drug whose mechanism is different.

Parkinson Caused by Drugs — Permanent Parkinson

In 1982 a man in California made and distributed MPTP, a narcotic-like drug. This was used instead of heroin by a large number of young addicts, several of whom developed PD. Dr. William J. Langston identified MPTP as the drug that caused selective damage to the substantia nigra, a damage that mimicked PD. Unlike the neuroleptics, MPTP-related PD did not disappear when MPTP was stopped.

As many as 400 addicts may have injected themselves with MPTP. While several developed mild PD symptoms, seven developed moderate-to-marked PD. These seven reported that shortly after shooting-up they noticed a burning sensation along the needle track, followed by a "high," followed by bizarre visual changes including hallucinations. They then had generalized jerking movements, and one had twisting postures of his arms, legs, and neck. Within a few days, all drooled, moved slowly, trembled, and spoke softly. Within two weeks all had advanced PD. Symptoms included bradykinesia, rigidity, resting tremor, and postural instability. Other symptoms included stooped posture, a shuffling gait, micrographia, loss of associated movements, masked facies, and freezing. None of the patients had dementia; all responded to Sinemet; and all, in time, developed complications including on and off, and dyskinesias.

Drugs cause Parkinson. By blocking the dopamine receptors neuroleptics cause a temporary PD-like disorder, one that disappears after the drug is stopped. MPTP and related chemicals enter the dopamine cells of the substantia nigra and damage the cells' machinery inside. This results in permanent PD such as what happened to the seven addicts in California. In idiopathic PD, the process that destroys the dopamine cells leaves the Lewy body; in MPTP Parkinson, MPTP doesn't leave a calling card. MPTP is now used to make a model of PD in monkeys, a model that has enabled doctors to better understand idiopathic PD and to devise new and improved treatments for PD.

Parkinson Caused by Manganese and Other Metals

Manganese is the twelfth most common element on earth and the fourth most widely used metal. It is used in the manufacture of steel and batteries. Potassium permanganate, a manganese salt, is used for bleaching fabrics, printing, dyeing wood, tanning leather, and water purification. Potassium permanganate can also be a source of manganese poisoning.

Manganese poisoning was first described in 1837 in five people who worked in a manganese ore-crushing plant and developed Parkinson symptoms. Parkinson symptoms have subsequently been described in others exposed to manganese. The onset of symptoms differs among miners and industrial workers and this probably reflects how the miners or workers are exposed to manganese. Miners inhale dust filled with manganese, resulting in psychiatric symptoms such as irritability, emotional instability, delusions, and hallucinations. These symptoms may last as long as one to three months after the miners leave the mine. This could result from manganese particles in the dust gaining access to the brain through the nose. The psychiatric symptoms are followed, after a variable period of time, by symptoms of Parkinson.

Industrial workers may absorb manganese containing chemical compounds through their skin, through their noses by inhaling, or through their mouths by accidentally swallowing them. Because the manganese in industrial plants is in a chemical form it is more easily absorbed by the body than manganese in dust. In industrial workers, unlike miners, the onset of Parkinson symptoms is not preceded by psychiatric symptoms. Headaches and muscle weakness (as distinct from slowness) are more prominent in manganese poisoning than in PD, as are cerebellar symptoms (similar to those in multiple system atrophy). Neck, limb, and trunk dystonia accompanied by painful cramps are more prominent than in PD. People poisoned by manganese often have a peculiar walk — they walk like a swaggering rooster. Dementia is frequent. Symptoms progress in many people even after withdrawal from exposure to manganese. Sinemet, dopamine agonists, and anticholinergic drugs have a variable effect.

On post-mortem examination, manganese poisoning results in nerve cell loss and scarring in the globus pallidus. The globus pallidus is the target to which the dopamine cells in the striatum project. It acts as a "brake" in the brain. Partial destruction, or non-selective destruction, as in manganese poisoning, locks the brake, slowing movement, and results in Parkinson symptoms. Selective destruction, or stimulation of the globus pallidus through deep brain stimulation, releases the brake and relieves Parkinson symptoms.

Other metals can damage the brain. Copper can cause symptoms similar to manganese. Copper poisoning occurs in Wilson disease, an inherited disease. In Wilson disease the normal amounts of copper in the diet accumulate and damage the liver and globus pallidus. Mercury poisoning occurs in miners exposed to liquid mercury, and in industrial workers exposed to mercury in chemical compounds. Mercury poisoning results in damage to the cerebellum, with symptoms different from those of copper or manganese poisoning. Sodium, potassium, calcium, and magnesium are the common metals in the body; accumulations or deficiencies of these metals cause a variety of symptoms, but rarely Parkinson.

Metals such as manganese, copper, and mercury can damage the brain. They do not, however, seek out the dopamine cells of the substantia nigra. Iron is found in high concentrations in the substantia nigra of people with PD. Iron is a vital metal and is normally found in the brain. Whether the high concentration of iron in the substantia nigra of people with PD is a cause or a result of PD is under study. This does not mean, however, that iron in the diet causes PD, or that iron, if needed, should not be taken.

Parkinson Caused by Carbon Monoxide and Other Chemicals

Carbon monoxide is a common, colorless, odorless gas that can cause brain damage. About 2% to 25% of people poisoned with carbon monoxide, poisoned to the point of going into a coma, die. Among people who go into a coma but recover, 2% to 40% develop symptoms. The severity of symptoms depends on the amount of carbon monoxide to which they were exposed, the duration of their exposure, and the severity and duration of their coma. It is not known if exposure to small amounts of carbon monoxide over a long period of time can damage the brain. Such exposure includes almost everyone in an industrialized country. It is thought that such exposure to carbon monoxide does not cause brain damage because the body has ways of detoxifying small amounts of carbon monoxide.

Some people poisoned by carbon monoxide remain in a coma with symptoms similar to those of others in a coma. Brain damage from a coma, regardless of the cause, is related to the degree of damage from a lack of oxygen at the level of the cell. In people who recover from a coma induced by carbon monoxide, some already have Parkinson symptoms and some develop Parkinson symptoms several days or weeks later. The Parkinson symptoms are similar to idiopathic PD. Dystonia resulting in unusual postures of the hands, feet, and trunk is more common in carbon monoxide Parkinson. Mood swings, aberrant behavior, confusion, memory loss, anxiety, and depression are common. The Parkinson symptoms, the dystonia, and mental changes may stabilize or progress. The Parkinson symptoms may not respond to Sinemet, dopamine agonists, or anticholinergic drugs.

At post mortem the changes in the brain resemble those of lack of oxygen, not PD. The changes, like the changes in manganese poisoning, are in the globus pallidus. Carbon monoxide enters the blood from the lungs and binds to the hemoglobin that is carried by red blood cells, thereby replacing the oxygen that is normally carried by hemoglobin. This results in all tissues and cells of the body experiencing a lack of oxygen. Some cells, such as those in the globus pallidus, are more sensitive to the lack of oxygen than other cells. This explains why the globus pallidus is more likely to be damaged by carbon monoxide.

Parkinson Caused by Cyanide

Cyanide fumes inhaled through the nose, or cyanide capsules swallowed into the stomach, result in dizziness, headaches, convulsions, and coma within minutes. The death rate is 95%. Among people who recover, 50% develop Parkinson symptoms. As in carbon monoxide poisoning, dystonia and mental changes are common. Cyanide, like manganese and carbon monoxide, damages the globus pallidus. However, the way cyanide damages the globus pallidus is different. Every cell in the body has its own energy source. The energy source is the mitochondria, structures inside the cell that act like storage batteries. Cyanide poisons the mitochondria resulting in damage to the cells. The cells of the globus pallidus are especially vulnerable to such damage.

Many different chemicals, such as gasoline and fuel additives, fungicides, herbicides, insecticides, and pesticides, are suspected of causing PD, although nothing has been proven. Some may act like neuroleptics, some like MPTP, some like manganese, some like carbon monoxide, and some like cyanide. Discovering which chemical, if any, causes Parkinson and how it does so will lead to a greater understanding of PD.

Why Do Fewer Women Have Parkinson Disease?

Women, by a ratio of 45 to 55, are afflicted less by PD than are men. This difference is more striking before the onset of menopause. Why? Doctors at Yale University, a National Parkinson Foundation Center of Excellence, have shown that estrogen has a protective effect on dopamine cells in the substantia nigra. In female monkeys if the dopamine cells are deprived of all estrogen, 30% of them die. This also shows that not all the dopamine cells need estrogen. If all the dopamine cells needed estrogen, then even more men would get PD. For the symptoms of PD to appear, at least 60% of the dopamine cells in the substantia nigra must be lost. If 30% of the dopamine cells in a woman are vulnerable to withdrawal of estrogen, then estrogen replacement after the onset of menopause may play a role in protecting them from PD. Doctors caution, however, that the findings are not sufficiently established to recommend estrogen replacement as a means of protecting against PD. The study does show how increasing knowledge of hormones will change the treatment of PD.

Do Environmental Chemicals Cause Parkinson Disease? Does Where You Live Matter?

Many doctors believe the cause of PD will be found in the environment — an as yet unknown chemical, toxin, or pollutant that results in an accelerated loss of the dopamine cells in the substantia nigra. Other doctors believe the cause is genetic, and most believe it is a combination of a chemical in the environment, an MPTP-like agent, and genetic factors.

To illustrate why some doctors think an environmental chemical may be a cause of PD, several surveys have shown that PD is more common in some regions than others. The National Parkinson Foundation conducted a simple study. Pharmaceutical companies track the sales of drugs, including Sinemet. From these data they can tell how many people are on Sinemet in each city, county, state, and zip code. As Sinemet is used almost entirely for PD, the NPF constructed a chart using this information (Figure 6.1). For each of the 50 states and the District of Columbia, the chart shows the number of people on Sinemet as a percentage of the population.

From these data the average prevalence of PD for the United States as a whole (based on the number of people on Sinemet) is

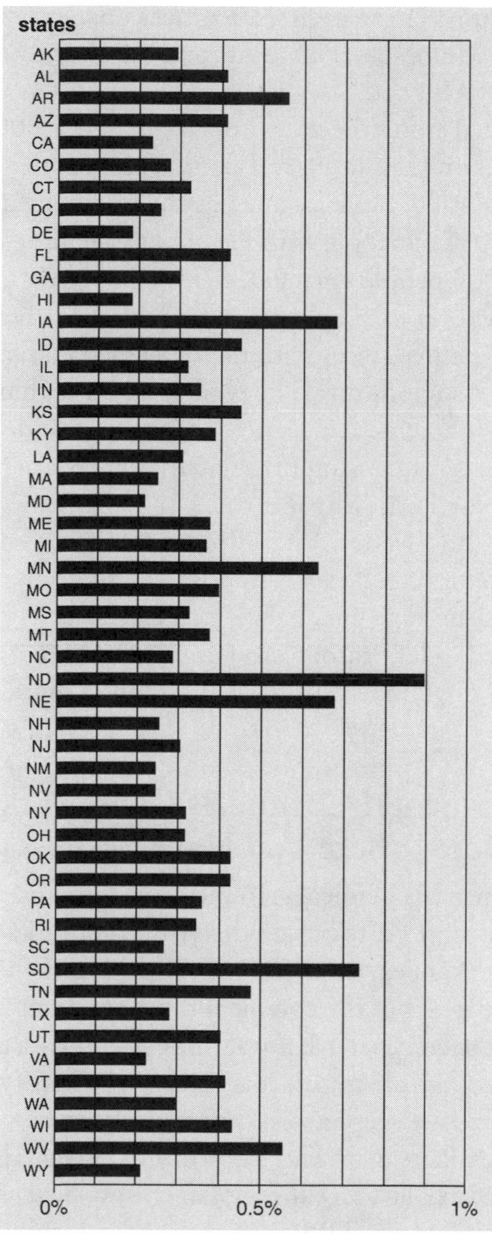

PD as a percent of the state's population ranges from a high in North Dakota of 0.9% of the state's population to a low in Hawaii of 0.18% of the states population.

Figure 6.1 *Prevalence of Parkinson Disease in the U.S. by State*

one person with PD for each 250 Americans, except in the five states of Iowa, Minnesota, Nebraska, and North and South Dakota, where the rate is higher.

In the United States there are approximately 1,000,000 people with PD based on the number of people on Sinemet in a population of 270,000,000. If we assume, as the pharmaceutical companies do, that 70% of people with PD are on Sinemet, then there are about 1,400,000 people with PD.

If the data are confirmed, this information can help to find the cause of PD. The five states with the presumed high prevalence of PD are rural and agricultural. They have a higher than normal use of fertilizers, fungicides, insecticides, and pesticides — all substances suspected of causing PD. The five states are populated by peoples of Northern Europe ancestry — Danes, Germans, Norwegians, and Swedes. Literally thousands of environmental and genetic factors can be superimposed on these areas of high PD prevalence to determine which ones may cause PD. Such factors can then be studied in laboratory models of PD to see if they accelerate the loss of dopamine cells in the substantia nigra.

Do Environmental Chemicals Cause Parkinson Disease? Does Where You Have Been Matter?

If an environmental chemical is found to be the cause of PD, exposure to it must start years before the symptoms of PD appear. The symptoms of PD appear after 60% of the dopamine cells in the substantia nigra die — but the chemical must start acting a long time before. And it becomes hard, if not impossible, 10, 20, or 30 years later to identify the chemical. It was easy to identify encephalitis as a cause of post-encephalitis Parkinson because all the people who developed Parkinson had a history of encephalitis. And it is easy to identify MPTP as a cause of Parkinson, because all the people who developed MPTP Parkinson had a history of injecting themselves with MPTP. Many soldiers suffered from exposure to Agent Orange during the Vietnam War. The veterans exposed to

Agent Orange were not examined after they were exposed. And now, as some develop PD, it is impossible to tell if their PD is related to Agent Orange or it is idiopathic. A recent event in which people were exposed to a number of chemicals is the Gulf War. Hopefully the veterans of the Gulf War will be followed more closely than the Vietnam veterans exposed to Agent Orange.

The Gulf War Syndrome and Parkinson (From an Article in the *NPF Parkinson Report*)

Up to 100,000 of 700,000 soldiers, sailors, airmen, and women who served in the Persian Gulf during operations Desert Shield and Desert Storm in 1990–1991 have complained about various symptoms that have been called the Gulf War Syndrome. Symptoms include memory loss, balance difficulty, sleep disturbances, depression, exhaustion, fatigue, and difficulty concentrating. Doctors examining veterans who have been diagnosed with Gulf War Syndrome are puzzled. Some doctors say there is no Gulf War Syndrome; the symptoms the veterans complain of are related to a post-traumatic stress disorder related to service during war-time. Other doctors say there *is* a Gulf War Syndrome, the symptoms being caused by a specific chemical, toxin, or virus the veterans encountered while serving in the Persian Gulf. If the symptoms are caused by contact with or exposure to a specific chemical, toxin, or virus the question arises — what are the long-term consequences of such contact or exposure? Could such contact or exposure result in PD? The question is not far-fetched. Five years ago the NPF proposed to the Department of Defense a detailed, long-term investigation of veterans suffering from Gulf War Syndrome to determine if these veterans were at increased risk for developing PD. The NPF's proposal was rejected. At the time it was judged there was insufficient evidence — other than the veteran's symptoms — of damage to the brain, to warrant such an expensive investigation.

On November 30, 1999, the results of a new study of Gulf War veterans were announced. The study was conducted by two renowned doctors, James Fleckenstein and Robert Haley of the

University of Texas Southwestern Medical Center in Dallas. The study used a technique called magnetic resonance spectroscopy to examine, in life, the chemical composition of the brains of veterans who served in the Gulf War. One group of veterans suffered from Gulf War Syndrome and a second group did not. Although the two groups were small, the differences between them were striking. The veterans who suffered from Gulf War Syndrome had lower levels of a specific chemical, abbreviated NAA, a chemical involved in energy metabolism. The lower levels of NAA, according to the doctors, indicated the loss of brain cells in the brainstem and basal ganglia — the areas targeted in PD.

A long-term study of veterans with Gulf War Syndrome would determine if they are more at risk for PD and would shed light on whether chemicals and toxins cause PD.

In Some People Parkinson Disease Is Inherited — Sometimes

Parkinson disease results from a loss of dopamine cells in the substantia nigra. In PD, but not the PD-like diseases, the loss of cells is associated with Lewy bodies. Lewy bodies are large, relative to the cell. Lewy bodies, as seen under the microscope, are made up of a dense core of particles surrounded by a rim of radiating fibers. Lewy bodies are associated with accumulations of three proteins: alpha-synuclein, parkin, and ubiquitin.

In 15% of people with PD, there's a family history of PD. PD may affect one or more members of a single generation, such as a brother and a sister. Or it may affect members of two generations, such as a mother and a son. It is impossible to say whether PD is hereditary, whether it is related to a chemical to which both family members were exposed, or whether it is chance. A way of determining if PD is hereditary is to study it in identical twins. A study done through the Veteran's Administration (VA) of identical twins revealed no difference in the occurrence of PD after age 60, but an increase in the occurrence of PD before age 50. This suggests heredity is important in people with young onset PD.

In about one half of one percent of people with PD, PD is strictly hereditary. In several American and European families a mutation on chromosome-4 results in PD and they develop PD before age 40. Otherwise their symptoms and response to medication are similar to typical PD. At post mortem the substantia nigra of these people, like people with typical PD, have a loss of dopamine cells associated with Lewy bodies. In several Japanese families a mutation on chromosome-6 results in PD and they develop PD under age 20. Otherwise their symptoms and response to medication are similar to typical PD. At autopsy these patients show a loss of dopamine cells not associated with Lewy bodies.

Genes are the blue print of the body's proteins. They are in a protected area of the cell called the nucleus and never leave it. Everyone has about 100,000 genes, entwined, like steel coils on 23 paired chromosomes (a total of 46 chromosomes). In everyone, each cell contains the full complement of 100,000 genes. However, each cell, or group of cells, is programmed to activate only a specific number of its 100,000 genes. The specific number of genes activated vary with the cell. Thus brain cells activate a different number of genes from liver cells. This results in brain cells producing different proteins from liver cells.

Genes consist of long strings of chemicals called DNA bases, arranged like beads on a necklace. There are four different types of DNA bases (the beads). The order in which the DNA bases follow each other has a meaning like the order in which letters follow each other to make a word. In the case of DNA, the meaning is an amino acid, and ultimately a protein. Each gene writes or transcribes its information onto RNA, a moveable molecule. The information written or transcribed onto RNA is then translated into proteins. Each gene codes for a single protein.

Proteins are made in or near the nucleus. After they are made, they are modified (or shaped) in two other regions. The relationship of one amino acid to *the one behind it* and the one *ahead* of it (the one-dimensional structure of the protein) is determined by DNA. Genetic defects or environmental chemicals may change the sequencing of amino acids. This, in turn, may change the protein's function. The 2-dimensional and 3-dimensional structure of each protein, its configuration in space, is determined after its amino acid sequence is laid down. When this is done the protein can finally start its work, for example housekeeping, or signaling, or transporting. Chemicals from outside or inside the cells may change the 2-dimensional or 3-dimensional shape of the protein.

Three Proteins Are Important in PD

1. Alpha-synuclein occurs in a restricted number of brain cells, including dopamine cells in the cortex and substantia nigra. Alpha-synuclein migrates from the nucleus through a series of hollowed-out tunnel-like structures or tubes (called fibrils) to the perimeter of the cell. Here, alpha-synuclein becomes associated with a specific kind of particle that stores dopamine. In PD, an abnormally shaped alpha-synuclein becomes stuck in one of the "tunnels." This build-up of alpha-synuclein becomes part of the Lewy body.
2. Parkin occurs in a restricted number of brains cells, including dopamine cells, in the cortex and brainstem. Parkin is made inside the cell's nucleus, from where it migrates through a series of "tunnels" to where it is needed. Parkin is a scavenger protein, one that breaks up abnormal clumps of other proteins (like alpha-synuclein). In PD, parkin, like alpha-synuclein, becomes misshapen and clumps on Lewy bodies.
3. The ubiquitins are a family of proteins that occur throughout the brain. They're ubiquitous — hence the name ubiquitin. Ubiquitins account for 2% of all brain proteins. The ubiquitins are formed inside the nucleus and migrate through the "tunnels" to where they are needed. The ubiquitins are scavenger proteins. In PD, the ubiquitins become misshapen and

accumulate on Lewy bodies. The accumulation probably results from an attempt by ubiquitins to break up the accumulation of alpha-synuclein.

Proteins that are not defective from birth may become defective because of aging. As proteins age, they slowly become damaged (oxidated) and toxic to a cell. Defective and damaged proteins are chopped up in the cell by a degrading engine. Proteins that have reached the end of their working lives are tagged by ubiquitin. They are then transported to the degrading enzyme, where they are chopped up into amino acids that are recycled for the formation of new proteins. If the tagging protein, ubiquitin, is itself defective, then instead of the protein being chopped up, it clumps and damages the cell.

Understanding how proteins become defective or damaged holds the key to understanding and curing PD and the PD-like disorders. Why do so many things cause Parkinson? To what end? To what good? In time we will know — and benefit. Isaiah wrote:

Who measured the water of the sea in the hollow of His Hand?
And calculated the Heavens to the nearest inch?
Gauged the dust of the earth to the nearest bushel?
Weighed the mountains on His scales?
And the hills on His balance?
Who but God.

CHAPTER

7

Parkinson and Anxiety

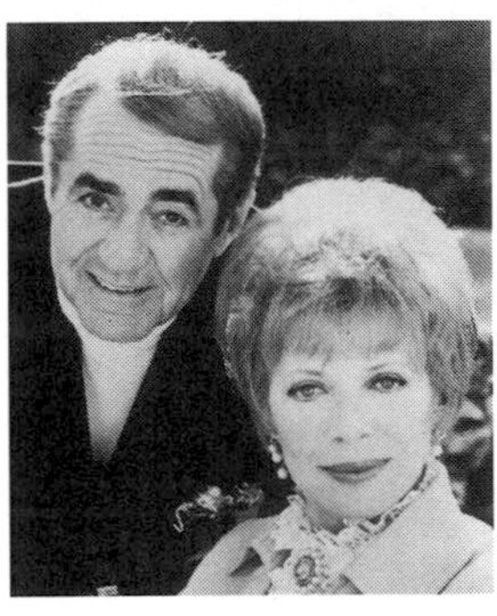

Henny Backus,
Actress, author of "Care for the Caretaker," wife of Jim Backus

"I was only 69 and very strong when Jim got sick. I still felt well when he died 11 years later. Somehow when I had to do it, I found the strength.

"How did I get him up and down the stairs? Going down stairs I walked in front of him – backwards. Going upstairs, I had to walk behind him.

"It was good for him to go out, good for him to face the world. If we knew we were going out to a restaurant, I would call ahead and ask them to have someone outside the front door at a certain time to help Jim out of the car and into the restaurant. Inside the restaurant, I cut his food for him—unobtrusively so I didn't embarrass Jim.

"Believe me, you will learn how to do everything all by yourself."

What Is Anxiety? Is It Good or Bad?

Anxiety is everywhere. All around us. It's universal. At different times, various words are used to convey the feeling of anxiety. Words commonly used as substitutes for anxiety include: afraid, fearful, stressed, tense, uncertain, worried, and terrified. Each conveys a different shade of meaning but it is the same feeling — one of anticipation or uncertainty, even of foreboding or fear. The words used to convey the feeling of anxiety vary from culture to culture, from language to language. And often, anxiety is expressed not in words but in physical symptoms such as feeling short of breath, dizzy, feverish, faint, restless, wobbly, or feeling your heart pounding.

How widespread is anxiety? Probably one-third of patients who visit a doctor, whether they are aware of it or not, do so solely because they are anxious. They may not know that the symptoms of feeling flushed, faint, jumpy, or tingling are part of anxiety. Untreated anxiety is an aggravating factor in many medical diseases, including PD.

Anxiety aggravates PD through the autonomic nervous system. (See Figure 4.1 on page 55.) During times of anger, fear, rage, or stress when the heart beats faster, blood pressure rises, hands shake more than usual, and the patient feels they are about to die — it is not PD; it is the autonomic nervous system, and it can be treated.

Approximately 54 million Americans — 20% — have an anxiety disorder as defined by the American Psychiatric Association and seek relief from anxiety by using prescription drugs. Approximately 81 million Americans — 30% — seek relief from anxiety by using legal, non-prescription drugs including alcohol or tobacco. But anxiety is not confined to hysterics, hypochondriacs, and neurotics. Most people in America and the world, knowingly or unknowingly, seek relief from anxiety in exercise, hobbies, school, work, and religion. The question is not are we anxious, but is our anxiety reasonable or unreasonable? Many with PD were anxious before PD. Parkinson does not lessen anxiety — it increases anxiety. And it makes it harder to tell how many symptoms are related to anxiety, to PD, or to the anxiety of having PD. And many who weren't anxious before developing PD became anxious when PD developed. In PD, the anxiety, if not understood and managed, can be more overwhelming than PD. This is shown by the following example:

Martha, a 48-Year-Old Woman Who Is Anxious

I was 45 years old when I noticed the tremor in my right hand. I work for a fashion magazine and beauty and glamour are important to me. I look at least 15 years younger than I am; I exercise regularly, I diet religiously, and I've had a face-lift. The tremor bothered me because my grandmother had Parkinson disease. But she was old — and I'm not. I'm divorced, three times, no children — thank you — and I date regularly. I prefer younger men; they're stronger, sturdier, less inhibited.

My friends say I'm affectionate, sensitive, sentimental, warm. My ex-husbands say I'm excitable, high-strung, temperamental — hysterical. And I admit I'm anxious. I've been in therapy since college. My therapist saw the tremor and referred me to a neurologist who diagnosed Parkinson. I don't know how I survived — but I did.

First I thought, maybe the neurologist's wrong and there's another reason for my tremor. So I had myself checked for low and high calcium, low magnesium, an underactive thyroid, and an overactive thyroid. Then, because of my love life, I had myself checked for syphilis and AIDS. Everything was normal. Then I had an MRI to rule out a stroke or a brain tumor. Then I got a second and a third opinion — both of which confirmed the diagnosis. I spent a year going from specialist to specialist and debating what to do.

By then my tremor had increased in frequency. Whereas before I could easily hide it by putting my hand in my pocket (I had taken to wearing slacks) now it was harder. I pleaded with the neurologist to stop the tremor. The next two years were an odyssey. I started with the anticholinergic drugs, the first drugs ever used for Parkinson. I went through Artane, Akineton, and Cogentin, singly and in combination. They helped, in part, but they made my mouth dry. They constipated me, and so bothered my bladder that I kept running to the bathroom. Next I tried Deprenyl. It helped, in part, but I became so hyper I couldn't sit still. Next, I tried several different tranquilizers. They helped, but I couldn't handle the side effects.

Then I tried the dopamine agonists: Mirapex, Permax, and Requip, singly and in combination. Each helped, in part, but each had a different side effect: dizziness, drowsiness, or swelling of my feet. And I gave up on them. Then I tried Sinemet and later, Sinemet and Comtan. These helped but I worried about using Sinemet at such an early stage. And although three neurologists reassured me, I stopped taking it.

Then I read about surgery. There are two types. In one they drill a hole in your brain. This releases a brake stopping the tremor. But there's a risk, under 1%, of stroke. I can't handle a tremor, I thought, how can I handle a stroke?

In the second operation, deep brain stimulation, they put a pacemaker in your brain, hook it up to a battery over your breast, and use a magnet to turn the pacemaker on and off. I turned deep brain stimulation down. What man, I thought, would sleep with a bionic woman?

The tremor was making me more anxious, and as I became more anxious, the tremor got worse. Then I met Jerry. He's a dentist and he's 10 years younger than me, but he didn't know it. He was going through a divorce — and he had a tremor. I could hide my tremor from him; he couldn't hide his tremor from me. One night, as we made love, his left hand shook so violently we had to stop. That's when he admitted he had Parkinson. I caressed him, comforted him, reassured him — but could not bring myself to tell him I had Parkinson. I broke off the relationship. He thought it was because he had Parkinson, not knowing it was because I had Parkinson. That was the beginning of my re-awakening, my coming to terms with Parkinson. I'm not religious, but a verse from the Bible, from Ecclesiastes, kept running through my brain:

VANITY OF VANITIES, ALL IS VANITY,
WHAT DO YOU GAIN FROM ALL YOUR TOIL?
A GENERATION COMES, AND A GENERATION GOES,
BUT THE EARTH GOES ON FOREVER.
THE SUN RISES, AND THE SUN SETS,

THE WIND BLOWS TO THE SOUTH, THE WIND BLOWS TO THE NORTH,
ROUND AND ROUND GOES THE WIND, AND RETURNS TO WHERE IT CAME.
AS THE EYE IS NOT SATISFIED WITH SEEING, NOR THE EAR WITH HEARING.
SO WHAT HAS BEEN IS WHAT WILL BE, AND WHAT HAS BEEN DONE IS WHAT WILL BE DONE.
THERE IS NOTHING NEW UNDER THE SUN.

My situation, my life, my PD is not unique, and I'll learn to deal with it. I recently took the Quality of Life Examination and did as follows:
My Mobility Index is 18 (out of 40 points).
My Emotional Index is 33 (out of 44 points).
My Autonomic Index is 7 (out of 16 points).
My Score on the Quality of Life Scale is 61%.
I consider my Quality of Life bad, but it will improve.

Mastering Anxiety by Measuring Anxiety

Think of anxiety as a fever: you feel warm, but unless you take your temperature, you do not know if you are abnormally warm. Similarly, you feel anxious — but until you measure your anxiety as you measure your temperature, you do not know how anxious you are. Are you normally anxious — like a normal temperature of 98.6 Fahrenheit? Or, is your anxiety level higher, like a fever of 101? To understand anxiety, a scoreboard — a thermometer — is needed and that is why the Anxiety Questionnaire was developed.

The questionnaire consists of 25 questions: 10 relate to words describing anxiety, 15 relate to the presence (or absence) of physical symptoms that accompany anxiety. The questionnaire is modeled on the Hamilton Anxiety Scale, the most widely used and studied scale and was developed over a 10-year period as a way of teaching patients, spouses, caregivers, and families of patients to identify, control, and master anxiety. By completing the questionnaire at different times and in various situations, you will determine how anxiety appears in you at these times. The questionnaire is a teaching aid; its statistical validity has not been established. The questionnaire complements the Quality of Life Examination.

THE ANXIETY QUESTIONNAIRE

Below are common symptoms of anxiety. Some may also be symptoms of PD, or side effects of the drugs used to treat PD. Regardless, if you are experiencing or have experienced a symptom in the past week please select "Yes," if not select "No."

1.	I feel my hands and/or feet tingling or burning.	Yes	No
2.	I feel flushed or feverish.	Yes	No
3.	I feel worried.	Yes	No
4.	I feel unsteady or wobbly.	Yes	No
5.	I feel nervous.	Yes	No
6.	I feel my vision is blurred.	Yes	No
7.	I feel anxious.	Yes	No
8.	I feel dizzy or lightheaded.	Yes	No
9.	I feel fearful or afraid.	Yes	No
10.	I feel I'm choking.	Yes	No
11.	I feel uncertain.	Yes	No
12.	I feel my hands and/or feet shaking or trembling.	Yes	No
13.	I feel I'm jumping or twitching.	Yes	No
14.	I feel I can't concentrate or pay attention.	Yes	No
15.	I feel my heart pounding.	Yes	No
16.	I feel insecure or I feel I'm losing control.	Yes	No
17.	I feel short of breath.	Yes	No
18.	I feel terrified.	Yes	No
19.	I feel my stomach's upset or I feel nauseated.	Yes	No
20.	I feel stressed or tense.	Yes	No
21.	I feel faint.	Yes	No
22.	I feel I'm sweating.	Yes	No
23.	I feel I'm panicked.	Yes	No
24.	I feel my ears ringing or buzzing.	Yes	No
25.	I feel hot or cold flashes.	Yes	No

If you answered yes to 15 or more questions, you are anxious and your anxiety must be addressed. Don't hide it; discuss it with your spouse, your family, and your doctor.

The Anxiety of Being Diagnosed with Parkinson Disease

If you were not anxious before you were diagnosed, you will be. If you do not know about PD, do not deny it or hide it; it will not go away. Find out as much as possible from reliable sources such as your doctor and the National Parkinson Foundation. If someone in your family has PD, do not assume what happened to them will happen to you. And do not assume they can give the advice you need. They could possibly be more anxious than you are and can increase your level of anxiety. Anna, the 57-year-old lady, was certain that she could not have PD because Parkinson was not in her plans. Because she knew she would be anxious when she saw the neurologist, she brought her daughter, a nurse, with her. Use your family for support. Because, like Anna, you are likely to be anxious when you see the doctor, you are likely to hear what you want to hear, not what the doctor said. A family member is more likely to hear what was actually said.

Jack, the 60-year-old handwriting expert whose father had PD, was terrified when after examining his own handwriting he diagnosed PD in himself. And he was certain he would become as "bad" as his father. If you are worried about what the future holds and the doctor does not mention this, you must. But if you say, "My father had PD and it was awful. Will I be as bad as my father?" you will probably not get a satisfactory answer, because words such as "awful" and "bad" do not mean anything concrete. The doctor will not know what you mean by "bad" and unless he took care of your father, he will not know how "bad" your father became. Before you see the doctor, in a calm moment, write down, precisely and unambiguously, what you fear the most. With Jack it was his voice. Jack's voice had changed and Jack was afraid that because after his father's voice had changed, his father had difficulty swallowing, the same thing would happen to him. The neurologist's explanation satisfied Jack and made him less anxious. The neurologist said that although the muscles of speech and swallowing are the same, they are controlled differently, and difficulty speaking does not necessarily mean difficulty swallowing.

Worrying About What Parkinson Will Do to Intimacy

Partners in loving relationships always look for ways to improve them. They are aware of each other's feelings and can spot signs of trouble. Loving relationships thrive because couples are willing to share. This is more true when one partner develops PD. Knowing how to talk to each other is the key to any relationship. Knowing how to talk means knowing how to listen. Think back to when you and your spouse met. Who started the conversation? Or maybe it started with a smile, a wink, or a nod. Couples who have been together a long time can read each other's minds. They know what the other is thinking. Do not let PD destroy the relationship. And, if for some reason you cannot get the words out, smile or nod. Do not be afraid to bring up forbidden topics. If you want to be intimate with your partner, do not think, "He's not interested in me anymore."

If you want to be intimate and your voice cannot say the words, leave a book on lovemaking or a provocative picture where he, or she, will find it. Be as seductive as you were on your honeymoon. The great silent film stars, the "vamps" of the 1920s — the Greta Garbos, the Gloria Swansons, the Rudolf Valentinos — were provocative and seductive without uttering a word. And, when you can, do not be afraid to say, "I'd like to make love to you."

Relationships are more than lovemaking. They are sharing and trusting. When Melvin, the state senator, was diagnosed with PD, he didn't want "to come out of the closet." He said, "Everyone knows me. I could be governor. So when I was diagnosed I told my staff and they said, 'Don't say anything. You'll never get elected.' My wife disagreed."

Later, Melvin said, "I ignored her advice and listened to my staff. My staff had a vested interest in my staying in office. My wife had a vested interest in doing what was best for us. I should have listened to her." Although Melvin and his wife disagreed initially, they always talked to each other and grew closer. When Melvin was asked to run for governor, he admitted he had PD, realized he would have problems, and turned to his wife. She ran and was elected.

Melvin and his wife find comfort in each other, and in the Bible. So can you.

If you want to serve God, prepare yourself for an ordeal.
Be sincere of heart, and do not be alarmed when danger comes.
Do not abandon yourself to sorrow, do not torment yourself with anger.

Many people with PD fear their spouse will no longer find them attractive. Having to deal with PD during your most intimate moments — when you have difficulty undressing yourself, when you have difficulty turning or positioning yourself in bed, or doing all of the things couples do to each other — is difficult. But these difficulties can be overcome or used to create new levels of respect and intimacy.

Physical attraction, despite the emphasis our culture places on it, is surface deep. This is illustrated by Martha who says,

". . . beauty and glamour are important to me. I look at least 15 years younger than I am. . . . my grandmother had Parkinson disease. But she was old — and I'm not. . . . I date regularly. I prefer younger men; they're stronger, sturdier, less inhibited."

To Martha, who's concerned with her appearance and wants to look young, having a tremor is devastating. But is it devastating because Martha has PD? Or because Martha's afraid of growing old like her grandmother? Addressing these fears, even if they sound silly, and talking about them leads to a resolution. Talking to each other brings couples together, makes them more sensitive and attractive to each other. Although Martha does not have a spouse to talk to, she, like you, can do many other things.

If, before you had PD, you paid attention to your looks, continue doing so. Clear up oily skin, find ways to stop drooling (it can be done), and if you tremble when you are excited, don't let it bother you. Remember if you tremble when you are exited, it reveals your feelings more than words. When you say, "I love you," and tremble, he knows you mean it. Listen to Martha when she's making love to Jerry, who also has PD. Each has not told the other they have PD: "I could hide my tremor from him; he couldn't hide his tremor from me. One night, as we made love, his left hand shook so violently we had to stop. That's when he admitted he had Parkinson. . . . I broke off the relationship. He thought it was because he had Parkinson, not knowing it was because I had Parkinson." How much better, how much closer would they have been, if each admitted they had PD, and each admitted the other "turned them on" anyway? Martha, by hiding her tremor, may have thought she was hiding her PD, but she was really hiding her passions — she did not trust anyone enough to be close to them.

Commit yourself, be truthful, and make time for intimacy and passion for these efforts are the cornerstones of a relationship. And, although Parkinson can challenge the most committed, intimate, truthful, and passionate couple, relationships endure and strengthen despite or because of PD. If, like Martha, you let PD become the central issue in your life, you will drive people away. Do not be a PD victim, be who you are — a person.

Listen to Anna who survived being diagnosed with PD and now, five years later, she and her husband are closer, more intimate. "Parkinson," says Anna, "is a warning, a red flag that you're mortal. Let it be what it is, a message from God:

For the heart of the wise is in the house of mourning,
But the heart of the fool is in the house of mirth.
It is better to hear the rebuke of the wise,
Then to hear the song of fools."

How Well Do You Know Each Other?

This self-examination, which complements the Quality of Life, may help you discover how well you know each other. You and your partner should take the examination. There are no right or wrong answers, only truthful answers.

1. The biggest change in our lives since I was diagnosed with PD is_______.

2. The biggest change in our relationship since I was diagnosed with PD is______.
3. The thing I fear most about PD is________.
4. The thing I love most about you is_______.
5. The most stressful thing about PD is______.

Ways of Reducing Anxiety

The Four Rs of Reducing Anxiety

One way of reducing anxiety is to avoid situations that cause anxiety. Unfortunately, many anxiety-provoking situations cannot be avoided, so you'll need to find ways to cope with the situation. Start with the "Four Rs of Coping":

Reorganize: One way of reducing anxiety is to reorganize your life. Jerry, the dentist, gave up his free-wheeling lovelife; Melvin, the state senator, let his wife run for governor.

Rethink: A second way of reducing anxiety is to re-think your priorities. Anna changed her responsibilities at work; Jerry hired an associate.

Relax: A third way of reducing anxiety is to find relaxation in exercise, hobbies, and meditation. These are discussed later.

Release: A fourth way is to become involved in something greater than yourself. Lenny, the man with Shy Drager, started a support group; Anna turned to the Bible.

Meditation

There are many methods, schools, and techniques of meditation. Through a process of trial and error, you will find the technique that best suits you. A simple method is to sit in a quiet room, or in a meadow away from the noise of crowds, and think of a calming image. Or, sit in a comfortable position and breathe in a calm, effortless way. Slow down your racing thoughts. Focus your attention on one thing. Chant, if it helps to focus your attention. Prayer is the most calming meditation of all.

Such techniques help turn off your sympathetic nervous system, the emergency button that prepares you for flight or fight. And such techniques help to turn on your parasympathetic nervous system: slowing your breathing, slowing your heart beat, relaxing your muscles, and reducing your anxiety.

Dealing with the Anxious People in Your Life

Some people, even family and friends, make you anxious. Such people, consciously or subconsciously, project their anxieties on you. Would you want to go on a date with Jerry? Or Martha? They may be good company but in a sexually charged situation they succeed in "projecting their anxieties on you," making you anxious, too.

Recognize the person who is making you anxious. Listen to what they are saying about you, because they are really talking about themselves. To tone down an argument set a rule: "You speak first and uninterrupted for as long as you want. Then I speak uninterrupted for as long as I want."

Be slow to anger. Remember, if one of you dies, and you haven't made peace with each other, the ensuing depression will be worse than the present anxiety. If you are becoming anxious, step back, sit in a comfortable position, and breathe in a calm, effortless way. Quiet your mind, slow down your thoughts. Then say, in as calm a way as possible, "You're making me anxious. Am I making you anxious?" If the answer is "Yes," be prepared to listen in silence. If you are not prepared to listen, do not ask the question.

Counseling

Although for most people, most of the time, it is the situation that sets the degree of anxiety, in certain situations some people are more likely to be anxious than others. Level of anxiety can be related to:

- Psychological makeup
- The chemistry of your brain
- Belief (or non belief) in God

Psychological makeup is set, in part, by the following:

- The order of your birth in relation to your sisters and brothers
- The absence of sisters and brothers (you're an only child)
- The relationship between your mother and father
- The relationship between you and your mother and father
- The relationship between you and your sisters and brothers
- The religious belief (or non belief) of your parents
- Your religious training and upbringing
- Your early development
- A major childhood trauma, such as the illness or death of a parent, the divorce or separation of your parents, a childhood illness, or a major change in your family's circumstances such as moving from one country to another
- Your school experience, including the presence of an influential coach or teacher
- An unrecognized learning or psychological problem, including attention deficit disorder, depression, or dyslexia
- Your experiences as an adolescent
- A major societal change, such as a depression, a famine, or a war

If your psychological makeup plays a major role in making you anxious, psychological counseling is helpful. Counseling can be short- or long-term. The type and length of counseling depends on your psychological makeup, the presence of a definable problem, and the background and training of the counselor or therapist. The goal of counseling is to provide insight into those factors, conscious and subconscious, that in a specific situation make you anxious.

Exercise

Exercise, or more precisely repetitive exercise, should be done daily for an hour each morning before the stress of the day begins. And, if necessary, should be repeated for an hour in the evening if the day has been unusually stressful. Repetitive exercises may include: riding a stationary or regular bicycle, running in place or on a treadmill, jogging, rowing, swimming laps, and walking. Such repetitive activity serves to relax a stressed and overactive sympathetic nervous system.

Breathing Techniques

Learning techniques to control your breathing is an important part of managing stress. Proper breathing relaxes your sympathetic nervous system by preventing hyperventilation. And proper breathing stimulates your parasympathetic nervous system, the calming response. Learning proper breathing techniques requires an understanding of how we breathe and what causes us to breathe abnormally.

How Anxiety Changes Your Breathing

During anxiety, fear, uncertainty, and worry cause you to breathe faster and, as a result, the levels of expired gas (carbon dioxide) in your blood drop. This further increases the rate of breathing. And it shifts breathing from the lower part of your lungs, the diaphragm, to the upper part of your lungs. You breathe from your chest instead of your belly. The diaphragm is a skirt-like muscle that separates the chest from the belly. When the lower lungs fill with air, they push on the diaphragm making the belly protrude. In belly or diaphragm breathing each breath is slower, deeper, and more efficient; you spend less energy on the mechanisms of breathing. In chest breathing, or hyperventilation, breathing is faster, shallower, and less efficient. You spend more energy on the mechanics of breathing.

Breathing Fast (Over-Breathing) or Hyperventilation

If you exercise fast, your heart pumps harder and faster, your blood circulates faster, and you breathe faster; you hyperventilate — some people with PD normally hyperventilate. You take in more oxygen, use the oxygen to burn sugar and fat, and generate energy and waste products in the form of acid and carbon dioxide (from burning sugar and fat). Because the heart pumps faster and the blood circulates faster, the carbon dioxide generated goes into solution (in the blood) and neutralizes the acids generated. The levels of carbon dioxide remain normal. If, however, you stop exercising, but force yourself to breathe fast, or over-breathe, your heart does not pump harder and your blood does not circulate faster. The carbon dioxide generated does not go into solution but is exhaled through the lungs. This results in increased excitability of the nerve endings in the mouth, hands, and feet resulting in tingling around the mouth and in the fingers and toes. This also results in blood vessels narrowing resulting in cold hands and feet, blurred vision, and ringing ears as blood is shunted away. Then the blood vessels inside the brain narrow, resulting in dizziness, or faintness, or difficulty with concentrating.

Controlling Anxiety by Controlling Hyperventilation

If you are anxious with or without PD and you hyperventilate, this will cause more anxiety. And if you are not anxious and you hyperventilate you will become anxious. Most people will normally breathe fast — hyperventilate — using their chest-wall muscles as a short-term response to many threatening or anxiety-provoking situations. Normally anxious people hyperventilate in most situations both threatening and non-threatening. Changing breathing from a fast chest-wall pattern to a slow, deep pattern of belly (or diaphragm) breathing can decrease anxiety.

As anxiety decreases so too will the physical symptoms associated with anxiety. High blood pressure can become normal, shortness of breath can disappear, the heart can stop pounding, and the numbness or tingling of mouth, fingers, and toes can disappear. If breathing can be changed to a pattern of belly breathing, the heart and blood vessels will be better protected, promoting long-term good health. Decreasing anxiety lessens the tendency to panic or fly into a rage.

How Can You Tell If You Are a Belly Breather?

Lay flat in bed looking up at the ceiling. Place your left hand over your chest. Place your right hand over your belly, your index finger in your belly button. This provides a strong cue to belly breathing. And subconsciously, it reminds you of life's most comfortable, least anxious place — your mother's womb. Breathe normally (for you) for one minute then ask:

1. Was your chest moving?
2. Was your belly moving?
3. Can't tell.

If the answer is two, congratulations, you are a belly breather. If the answer is three, you're a chest breather. Repeat the above test at different times, in various situations over at least a month to see if you are consistently a chest or belly breather. Take the Anxiety Questionnaire on each day of the month. Then look at the situations in which you are breathing from your chest or from your belly. It is likely you are more anxious on those days in which you are a chest breather. Situations in which to note whether you are a chest or a belly breather include:

1. Laying flat in bed, your face looking down at the bed. Here, pressure on your belly from the bed may cause you to breathe from your chest. Work at learning to breathe from your belly regardless of position.
2. Sitting, before eating. Here, low blood sugar acting through your sympathetic nervous system may cause you to breathe fast, from your chest. Work at learning to breathe from your belly regardless of how hungry you are.
3. Sitting, after eating. Here, a full belly may cause you to breathe fast, from your chest. Work at learning to breathe from the belly regardless of how full (or empty) it is. This may help to better digest food.
4. Sitting or standing before a fearful or stressful situation. A fearful or stressful situation may cause you to breathe fast, from your chest due to your sympathetic nervous system. This hyperventilation will, in turn, increase your fear or stress. Work at learning to breathe from your belly especially when you are fearful or stressed. This helps relieve the sympathetic nervous system and helps stimulate the parasympathetic nervous system. The fear or stress will not go away, but it will help you approach the situation reasonably, without panic or rage.
5. Sitting or standing after a fearful or stressful situation. After a fearful or stressful situation is over, you may expect that you would be calm, relaxed, at

> peace. But, in this situation, if you breathe from your chest you are not as calm as you think. Work at learning to breathe from your belly even if you are calm, relaxed, at peace — it will help you remain that way.

Chest breathers are more likely to breathe at rates of 18 breaths per minute or higher and are more likely to hyperventilate. By changing from a chest breather to a belly breather you can, in time, lower your blood carbon dioxide, and improve the tone of your blood vessels, including your heart. And you will be less likely to panic or fly into a rage.

How Can You Change from a Chest Breather to a Belly Breather?

If you are a chest breather lying down, sitting, or standing, start your training lying down. After you have mastered becoming a belly breather lying down you can go on to becoming a belly breather in almost every situation. Be aware of whether you are a chest or a belly breather. Most people do not realize they are chest breathers, do not realize they hyperventilate, and do not realize they are making themselves more anxious. To become a belly breather:

- Lay flat in bed, your legs straight.
- Put your left hand on your chest, your right hand on your belly, with your index finger in your belly button.
- Take a deep breath, through your nose.
- Make certain the inhaled air reaches the bottom of your lungs. You will know this because your diaphragm will move down forcing your belly against your right hand — pushing your index finger out of your belly button. And, subconsciously, perhaps disconnecting you from your umbilical cord.
- Hold the air in your lungs as long as you can, then exhale from your belly.
- Practice so that you consistently, every breath, breathe from your belly. Do this at least 60 times.

If in any situation, you are so anxious that you have difficulty breathing from your belly, cup both your hands over your nose and mouth and breathe into your cupped hands, breathing and re-breathing the expired air. This raises the carbon dioxide in the air you breathe and raises, temporarily, the carbon dioxide in your blood. This action calms and relaxes you by reversing, temporarily, the effects of hyperventilation.

Drugs: Changing the Chemistry of the Anxious Brain

The following is a description of the drugs that are available to treat anxiety. Many are the same drugs used to treat depression, difficulty sleeping, phobias, and panic attacks. This emphasizes the similarity in the chemistry of these conditions. Although the drugs may be the same, the following aspects may differ from condition to condition: the dosing of the drug (in milligrams) needed in a particular condition; the scheduling of the drug, such as the frequency and the time when it should be taken, and the combination of the drugs. (In a specific condition drugs from two or more categories may be used sequentially or simultaneously.)

The main naturally occurring chemicals in the brain regulating anxiety are Gamma Amino Butyric Acid (GABA), norepinephrine, and serotonin (Figure 7.1). The commonly used prescription drugs affect these chemicals. Such drugs, when they're used for difficulty sleeping, are likely to cause daytime grogginess or drowsiness.

The levels of the naturally occurring brain chemical GABA are affected by a class of drugs called *benzodiazepines*. The benzodiazepines bind to a receptor, a specific protein called the GABA-receptor, located on nerve cells in a specific region of the brain. This results in a calming effect. The benzodiazepines act within minutes to hours. Benzodiazepines do not cure anxiety, however they mask it like aspirin masks a fever. By calming you down, benzodiazepines allow you to deal with many anxiety-provoking situations later at a more favorable time. Benzodiazepines are used to treat anxiety, agitated depression, panic attacks, phobias, and rages. Some benzodiazepines, such as Klonopin and Valium, are also used to treat muscle spasms.

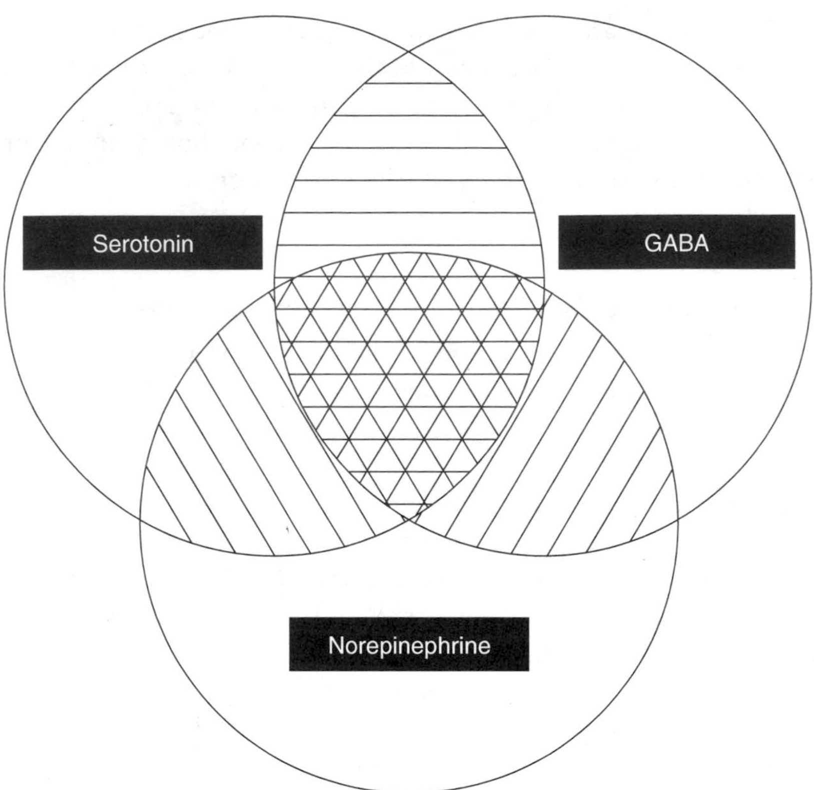

Figure 7.1 Treating Anxiety

Benzodiazepines can cause drowsiness and the labels contain warnings about driving or operating machinery. Side effects, especially in older people or intellectually impaired people, can include agitation (a paradox, as benzodiazepines are usually calming), confusion, delusions, hallucinations, memory loss, unsteadiness, and clumsiness. The side effects disappear after the drug has been stopped. A rule of thumb is that it may take as long as five half-lives for the drug to clear your system and the side effects to resolve.

The following list of benzodiazepines includes the drug's generic name, the drug's brand name, the usual nighttime dose in milligrams (mgs), the drug's time to peak onset (in hours) — a measure of how long it takes for the drug to have an effect, the drug's half-life (in hours) — a measure of how long the drug's effects last. Some drugs have a long half-life, reflecting delayed metabolism by the body.

Aprazolam (Xanax) Usual dose 0.25 mg, two to three times a day. Peak onset 1–2 hours. Half-life 6–26 hours. For difficulty sleeping, given as a single 0.25 or 0.50 mg dose at night.

Clonazepam (Klonopin) Usual dose 0.5 mg, two to three times a day. Peak onset 1–4 hours. Half-life 30–40 hours. For difficulty sleeping, given as a single 0.5 to 1.0 mg dose at night.

Diazepam (Valium) Used for anxiety, panic, muscle spasms, epileptic seizures. Usual dose is 2 to 5 mg, two to three times a day.

Lorazepam (Ativan) Usual dose 1 mg, two to three times a day. Peak onset 2 hours. Half-life 12–18 hours. For difficulty sleeping, given as a single 1 to 2 mg dose at night.

Temazepam (Restoril) Usual dose 15 mg. Peak onset 1.5 hours. Half-life 3–18 hours. Used exclusively for difficulty sleeping. Given as a single 15 to 30 mg dose at night.

Serotonin and the Selective Serotonin Re-uptake Inhibitors

The naturally occurring brain chemical serotonin acts as a messenger carrying information from one cell to another in specific regions of the brain. Serotonin is released by a specific cell and concentrates in the gap between the cell that released it and another cell. It tones down the excitability of both cells. The *selective serotonin re-uptake inhibitors* (SSRIs) block the re-uptake of serotonin, allowing it to concentrate in specific regions of the brain, resulting in an increased concentration outside the cells. This makes it less likely that the cells will be excited.

SSRIs are used to treat depression, phobias, panic attacks, obsessive compulsive disorders, and increasingly to treat anxiety. Although they may peak rapidly, they take two to four weeks to build up and change the chemistry of the brain. Because of their great effectiveness versus other drugs and their favorable side-effect profile they have become the chief means of treating these disorders.

Because SSRIs must build up, and are not as fast acting as benzodiazepines, a single dose of an SSRI will not stop or prevent a panic attack or calm an anxiety-provoking situation. Side effects, some of them seemingly contradictory, include apathy, agitation, decreased sex drive, dizziness on standing, delusions, difficulty sleeping, hallucinations, headaches, sweating, twitching, unsteadiness, weight gain, or weight loss. The side effects disappear after the drug has been stopped. But it may take as long as five half-lives for the side effects to completely resolve. SSRIs increase the effects of benzodiazepines and combinations of an SSRI and a benzodiazepine must be used with caution. SSRIs, like all drugs, work best when combined with counseling: both psychological counseling and spiritual counseling. Consider using SSRIs for Jack, Jerry, and Martha. SSRIs will not make them happy but might, initially, help them face their PD more calmly. SSRIs include:

Fluoxetine (Prozac) is used for depression, obsessive-compulsive disorders (a form of anxiety), phobias, and panic attacks. Prozac peaks at 4 to 8 hours. Its half-life is 48 to 215 hours. The usual dose is 20 to 40 mg once a day. Prozac is an "activating" drug. This makes it useful for treating an "apathetic" depression. Conversely Prozac may increase the agitation of an agitated depression.

Paroxetine (Paxil) is used for anxiety, depression, obsessive-compulsive disorders, phobias, and panic attacks. Paxil peaks at 5 hours. Its half-life is 21 hours. The usual dose is 10 to 40 mg once a day.

Sertraline (Zoloft) is used for anxiety, depression, obsessive-compulsive disorders, phobias, and panic attacks. Zoloft peaks at 5 to 9 hours. Its half-life is 25 to 65 hours. The usual dose is 50 to 100 mg once a day.

Other Drugs That Affect Chemicals in the Brain

Buspirone (Buspar) affects serotonin and dopamine. It is fast acting and is used in anxiety, obsessive-compulsive disorders, and panic attacks.

Beta blockers are drugs that block a specific receptor, a protein, found on the endings of sympathetic nerves or their target organs. By blocking the receptor the drugs prevent the nerves or the organs from responding to norepinephrine. In this way beta-blockers relax the sympathetic nervous system which in turn relieves many of the physical symptoms that accompany anxiety. Beta blockers can decrease trembling, restlessness, heart pounding, sweating, and hot flashes. They act rapidly and can prevent panic in anxiety-provoking situations. They are not addictive. In some people they cause or aggravate daytime drowsiness, insomnia, dizziness on standing, asthma, fatigue, depression, hallucinations, and memory loss. The most commonly used beta blockers are:

Propranolol (Inderal). It peaks in 60 to 90 minutes. Its half-life is 4 to 6 hours. It is used to treat the physical symptoms associated with anxiety, phobias, and panic attacks. Inderal enters the brain. This may, at times, be an advantage, because Inderal may block receptors in the brain that aggravate anxiety.

Atenolol (Tenormin) does not enter the brain. It is less effective than Inderal in treating certain symptoms associated with anxiety, phobias, and panic attacks. It may have fewer side effects. Consider using beta blockers for Jerry when he goes into his office.

When facing a disease like Parkinson, where anxiety increases and sleep is disrupted, do not forget the Bible. With the Bible's help and the help of science you will reach the state of which Isaiah dreamed:

When the eyes of the blind shall be opened,
And the ears of the deaf unstopped.
When the lame shall leap like a deer,
And the tongue of the mute shall sing for joy.
When waters shall break forth in the wilderness,
And streams in the desert.

When the wolf will live with the lamb,
And the leopard will lie down with the kid,
And when a little child will lead them.
When the lion shall eat straw like the ox,
When they will not hurt or destroy,
And when the earth will be full of the knowledge of God,
As the waters that cover the sea.

Difficulty Sleeping

Difficulty sleeping is discussed here because sleep disorder and anxiety go together: anxiety results in difficulty sleeping and difficulty sleeping results in anxiety. The treatment of one helps the other. Although difficulty sleeping is common in PD it is usually ignored or trivialized because difficulty sleeping is usually self-limited and without consequences. Difficulty sleeping in people with or without Parkinson may consist of one or more of the following:

1. Difficulty falling asleep
2. Difficulty remaining asleep
3. Frequent nighttime awakenings
4. Early-morning awakening
5. Un-refreshing sleep.

Temporary difficulty sleeping, affecting four or more nights each week for less than four weeks, is common and usually has no consequences. It occurs for no apparent reason in up to 50% of all people. Chronic difficulty affecting four or more nights each week for more than four weeks is less frequent. Such difficulty may have consequences such as daytime fatigue, grogginess, irritability, mood swings, and difficulty paying attention. Chronic difficulty sleeping, in people with or without PD, may be associated with other diseases including heart, lung, bladder, and prostate disease. If a person with PD has one of these other diseases, the other disease as well as the PD may aggravate the sleeping problem. Successful management of difficulty sleeping requires recognizing and treating both the PD and the other disease. People with chronic difficulty sleeping are more than twice as likely as people with normal sleep to suffer from (1) anxiety, (2) depression, (3) mood swings, and (4) delusions. Whether these conditions came first and chronic difficulty sleeping followed, or vice versa is a topic of serious debate and study.

Conditions Causing Difficulty Sleeping

Temporary difficulty sleeping may be caused or triggered by:

1. Anxiety and worry over family, friends, or business.
2. Situational adjustments including a new or strange bed, house, or room; a new job; or a new bed partner.
3. Changes in the normal sleep–wake cycle such as international jet travel or a change in work schedule, especially in people who work varied shifts.
4. A new drug, either a prescription or an over-the-counter drug.

People with temporary difficulty sleeping often try to correct the difficulty on their own, using such methods as relaxation techniques, herbal remedies, or over-the-counter drugs. If the difficulty sleeping persists, the person will likely see a doctor.

Most people who see a doctor because of difficulty sleeping have chronic difficulty sleeping. (Figure 7.2) Among the causes are:

1. Anxiety
2. Depression
3. Heart or lung disease that results in shortness of breath upon lying down
4. Kidney, prostate, or bladder disease that results in frequent nighttime awakenings to urinate
5. Disease of the stomach that results in acid reflux upon lying down
6. Endocrine disease such as overactive thyroid gland
7. Arthritis or any condition that causes pain

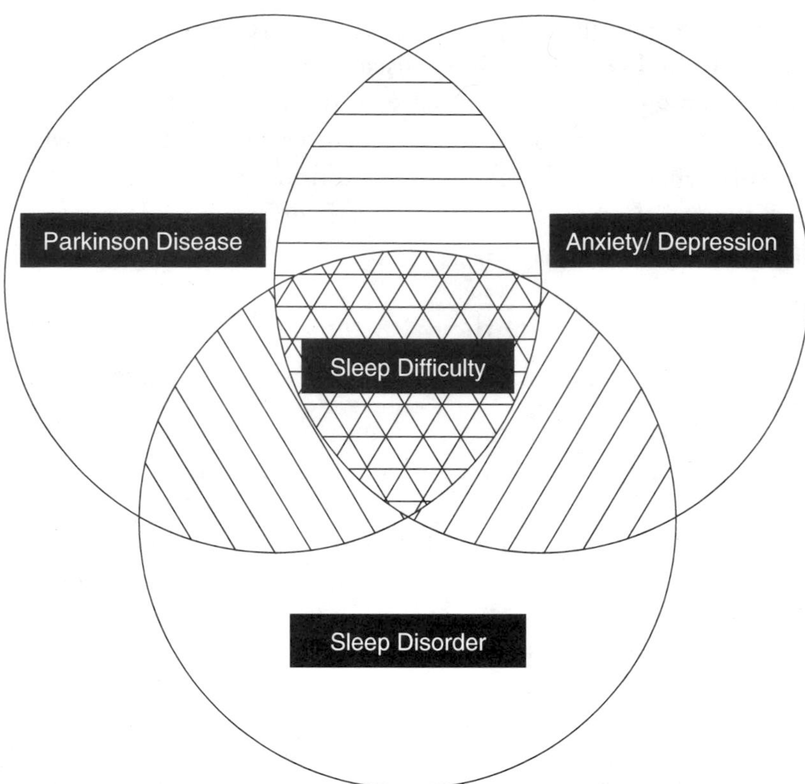

***Figure** 7.2 Main Causes of Sleep Difficulty in Parkinson Disease*

8. Drugs prescribed for all of the above conditions
9. Sleep apnea that results from laxness of the muscles of the roof of the mouth. This results in the uvula falling back into the throat and partially blocking the airway upon lying down.

Primary Sleep Disorders

Primary sleep disorders arise from an unknown disturbance in sleep rhythm. Primary sleep disorders account for perhaps 10% of all people with chronic difficulty sleeping. The centers regulating sleep are in the brainstem, which is uniquely positioned to regulate sleep, as it regulates eye opening and closing, posture, and tone. The major components of falling asleep — closing your eyes, relaxing your muscles, and adjusting to a lying down position — are regulated by the brainstem. The centers regulating sleep are located near the region primarily affected in PD. Thus, it is not surprising that there is an association between PD and difficulty sleeping.

The diagnosis of a primary sleep disorder, a disorder in 24-hour bodily rhythms, called "circadian rhythms," is made in the absence of other causes of difficulty sleeping, including all the conditions listed above. Sometimes, the diagnosis of a primary sleep disorder requires evaluation in a sleep laboratory. The most dramatic example of a primary sleep disorder and the association between PD and difficulty sleeping occurred during the epidemic of encephalitis that struck the world between 1918 and 1926. It is estimated that the epidemic affected 15 million people. During the initial infection, people experienced major difficulty sleeping including:

1. Falling into a deep sleep from which it was difficult to awaken.
2. Abruptly waking up, eating, drinking, and then falling asleep again.
3. Sleeping for many days without waking up.

So prominent and striking was the difficulty sleeping that another name for the encephalitis was "sleeping sickness." Upon recovery from the infection 40% of people who had encephalitis developed chronic difficulty sleeping. Among the patterns they showed were:

1. An inability to fall asleep
2. Frequent awakenings during the night
3. An inability to sleep more than two to four hours a night, staying awake until 4 A.M.
4. Sleeping till noon
5. Grogginess upon awakening
6. Napping during the day, often in inappropriate situations such as eating
7. Talking, crying out, or shouting during sleep

Upon recovery from encephalitis up to 40% of people developed PD. Many people developed both difficulty sleeping and PD. The most notable and infamous victim of encephalitis was Adolf Hitler.

Parkinson Disease and Difficulty Sleeping

People with early or recently diagnosed PD, people not on PD drugs, may have a variety of sleep difficulties. If the person with PD has difficulty sleeping and is not anxious or depressed, the difficulty sleeping may be related to rigidity and slowness of movement resulting in difficulty turning in bed. This difficulty sleeping may improve with PD drugs. These drugs, Sinemet plus Comtan, or a dopamine agonist that helps you turn in bed, allow you to sleep. If doubtful, try to fall asleep without changing position or turning in bed.

Up to 40% of people with early PD are anxious or depressed. Anxiety or depression will aggravate the difficulty sleeping. In people with PD who are anxious or depressed, the treatment of anxiety or depression will improve the difficulty sleeping. Selegiline (Deprenyl) may be used as a first treatment for PD. This may cause difficulty sleeping. Selegiline is often changed to amphetamine and in some people this causes difficulty sleeping. To minimize this, do not take selegiline after noon.

In some people with PD the difficulty sleeping is related to restless legs. See previous discussion.

People with advanced PD, on several PD drugs, may have a variety of sleep difficulties. Here the difficulty sleeping may be related to:

1. Difficulty turning or changing position in bed
2. Wearing off of PD drugs during the night
3. Restless legs
4. An effect of one or several PD drugs
5. Anxiety

6. Depression
7. A primary sleep disorder

If the difficulty sleeping is related to difficulty in turning in bed, wearing off of PD drugs during the night, or restless legs, treatment is the addition of Sinemet-CR plus Comtan, or a dopamine agonist at night. If the difficulty sleeping is secondary to an effect of the PD drug, then the addition of Sinemet or a dopamine agonist at night may aggravate the difficulty sleeping. Treatment is the addition of a sleep-promoting drug, but one that reverses the effects of the PD drug, a drug such as an atypical major tranquilizer such as Clozaril or Serequel. If the difficulty sleeping is related to anxiety, depression, or a primary sleep disorder the treatment is as outlined previously.

In addition, for many people with long standing PD, daytime drowsiness is a problem. They may or may not be aware of this. The cause of the daytime drowsiness in people with long-standing PD is usually

1. A selective decline in intellect
2. Dementia, a global decline in intellect
3. Depression

The decline in intellect may be associated with:

1. Hallucinations
2. Delusions
3. Agitation
4. Disinhibited or disruptive behavior, such as acting out

Selective decline in intellect or dementia may be part of advanced PD, secondary to involvement of brain regions necessary for thinking. Daytime drowsiness, hallucinations, delusions, agitation, and disruptive behavior result from the effects of anti-Parkinson drugs on an impaired brain. The difficulty sleeping at night worsens the daytime drowsiness. The difficulty sleeping at night in people with advanced PD is best treated with Clozaril and Serequel. Daytime drowsiness may respond, in part, to drugs such as Exelon, a drug used to treat the intellectual decline in Alzheimer disease. Daytime drowsiness does not usually respond to alerting drugs such as amphetamine that may aggravate hallucinations or delusions. Daytime drowsiness may respond to Provigil, a non-amphetamine alerting drug.

Evaluating Sleep

Prior to discussing treatment, the degree of difficulty sleeping at night should be measured. This can be done using a scale such as the one below.

NIGHTTIME SLEEP QUESTIONNARE

Evaluate yourself on a typical night. If you had difficulty sleeping the past week, answer the following:

1.	Did you take something for sleep?	Yes	No
2.	Did you go to bed after midnight?	Yes	No
3.	Did an hour or more elapse from laying down until falling asleep?	Yes	No
4.	Did you wake up, for any reason, more than once during the night?	Yes	No
5.	Did an hour or more elapse from laying down again until falling asleep?	Yes	No
6.	Did you wake up, for the last time, before 4 A.M.?	Yes	No
7.	Did you get less than four hours sleep per night?	Yes	No
8.	Did you get less than two hours sleep per night?	Yes	No
9.	When you woke up and got out of bed, were you groggy?	Yes	No
10.	Did you nap more than once per day?	Yes	No

If daytime drowsiness is a problem this should be evaluated using a scale such as the one below. This scale requires the cooperation of your spouse or care partner.

DAYTIME DROWSINESS

1.	Falls asleep before midday meal?	Yes	No
2.	Falls asleep during midday meal?	Yes	No
3.	Falls asleep before evening meal?	Yes	No
4.	Falls asleep during evening meal?	Yes	No
5.	Falls asleep while with company?	Yes	No
6.	Falls asleep while on the toilet?	Yes	No
7.	Falls asleep while watching TV?	Yes	No
8.	Falls asleep while riding in the car?	Yes	No
9.	Falls asleep when reading?	Yes	No
10.	Groggy while awake?	Yes	No

Treatment

Treatment of people with difficulty sleeping starts with finding the cause, evaluating the severity and then providing treatment. If difficulty sleeping is caused by a primary sleep disorder, treatment is to provide information about sleep and teach you about such simple and effective measures as:

- Going to bed only when you are sleepy
- Leaving your bedroom, if you're unable to fall asleep within 30 minutes, and returning only when you are sleepy
- Waking up at the same time every morning, including weekends
- Avoiding daytime naps

Certain relaxation techniques are useful in promoting sleep. Examples include neck muscle relaxation and belly breathing, discussed previously. Some people with difficulty sleeping try to compensate for their difficulty sleeping by engaging in activities that unknowingly aggravate the problem. Examples of such activities include excessive use of stimulants such as coffee or caffeinated soft drinks, drinking alcohol to promote sleep, sleeping excessively on weekends, and daytime napping. Many people with difficulty sleeping become anxious and preoccupied with their difficulty sleeping. And, as worry and concern tend to peak around bedtime, this worsens the problem.

If education about difficulty sleeping and instruction in proper sleep hygiene are insufficient, a second-line approach is the short-term use of a prescription or non-prescription drug. Commonly available prescription and non-prescription drugs are listed below. The proper drug, or combination of drugs, must be decided upon by you and your doctor.

Non-Prescription Drugs

These drugs, although not requiring a prescription, may have side effects and interactions with prescription drugs. You must tell your doctor of any and all sleep preparations you take.

Kava-kava root, usually up to 500 mg per night.

Melatonin, a hormone secreted by the pineal gland, thought to regulate circadian rhythms, usually 1 to 3 mg per night.

Valerian root, usually 500 mg per night.

Prescription Drugs

Non-Benzodiazepines are not benzodiazepines but bind to the same receptor. They are short acting, rapidly promote sleep, and rarely cause daytime drowsiness. They are less addicting than benzodiazepines. At present they are preferred as the short-term treatment for difficulty sleeping. They include:

Zolpidem (Ambien) Usual dose 5–10 mg. Peak onset 1.5 hours. Half-life 2–4 hours.

Non-Tri-Cyclic Antidepression drugs

These drugs are used to treat depression, but like tri-cyclic drugs, they may be used to treat difficulty sleeping in the absence of depression. They include:

Mirtazapine (Remeron) Usual dose 15 mg. Peak onset 2 hours. Half-life 20–40 hours.

Trazadone (Desyrel) Usual dose 50–100 mg. Peak onset 1–2 hours. Half-life 5–9 hours.

CHAPTER
8

Depression in Parkinson Disease

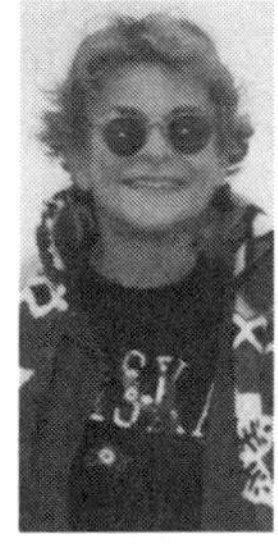
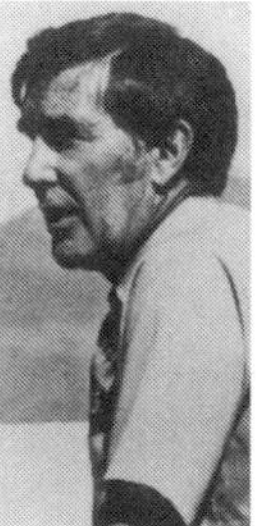

Norma Udall,
former lobbyist and wife of
Congressman Morris Udall

"Parkinson disease impacted my husband's career, and it impacted our marriage. But we accepted it together as a 'given.' Because I had known Mo for some years before we married, I often said, 'One of my eyes sees a man with an illness; the other eye sees that strong, splendid man who was so articulate and funny. He's the same Mo.'

"If I could make it easier for someone else, another wife or husband of a Parkinson patient, I'd say 'be proactive.' Get in there and be a part of it with him. Work with your spouse and against the disease. Fight it.

"Mo was a proud man, but he didn't allow the limitations of the disease to spoil his good times, nor did he ever complain. He put it out of his mind. We'd go out to dinner and it never bothered him if I cut his food or even sometimes had to feed him. If people noticed, it was unimportant to him.

"As a care partner, you want to make things as easy as possible for your spouse, but you must give him latitude to preserve his dignity. That is so important — for any of us. As the disease progresses and he requires more and more assistance for his daily needs, he must feel that he is in control of his own life. No matter how much you need to help him, he must never feel helpless.

"And though his muscles may not be responding to the instructions from his brain, and his face may not register emotions — we are aware, always, that there's an extraordinary human being — a person whom we love, still inside. And that is unchanged."

When Anna from Chapter 1 was diagnosed with PD and read about it, she became depressed. Her husband Bruce, and her daughter, Kathy, were her rocks — her support. Jerry, the dentist from Chapter 3, was going through a divorce when he was diagnosed with PD. He was depressed before he was diagnosed and without a support, he became more depressed. Jack Jr. from Chapter 2 never came to terms with his father, Jack Sr.'s PD and feared becoming like his father. As soon as Jack Jr. was diagnosed with PD, he became depressed. Martha from Chapter 7 was anxious before she was diagnosed with PD and became more anxious after she was diagnosed. Her anxiety, unless confronted and managed, will lead to depression. Lenny from Chapter 5 wasn't depressed when he was diagnosed with Shy Drager because his wife, Laurie, and God, are his rocks. Lenny and Laurie quote Isaiah:

> Did you not know?, Have you not heard?
> People grow tired and weary, They stumble and fall.
> But those who believe in God, Will regain their strength.
> They will sprout wings like eagles,
> And though they run, they will not grow weary,
> And though they walk, they will not tire.

The Depression Questionnaire

What is depression? Is depression normal in PD? And how do you know if you're depressed? Sometimes trying to decide if you're depressed, or if you have PD, or both, is difficult. Thus a PD person who has a sad, poker face, a soft, weepy voice, and a stooped posture (bent as though bearing the weight of the world on his shoulders) may appear depressed — when he's not. Conversely, a depressed person who moves slowly, speaks softly, and walks stooped over may appear to have PD when he does not. You may be depressed if during the past week you:

- Cried for no obvious reason.
- Felt sad, helpless, or guilt-stricken.
- Had difficulty sleeping at night or slept all day.
- Felt anxious, fearful, uncertain or worried for no obvious reason.
- Lost interest in your work, hobbies, family, or friends.
- Began drinking alcohol heavily.

The Depression Questionnaire modeled on the Hamilton Depression Scale may show if you're depressed.

DEPRESSION QUESTIONNAIRE

If during the past week, on four or more days, you had one of the following symptoms select "Yes," if not, select "No."

1.	I often felt sad.	Yes	No
2.	I often felt discouraged.	Yes	No
3.	I often felt blue.	Yes	No
4.	I often felt that I was a failure.	Yes	No
5.	I often felt upset.	Yes	No
6.	I often felt bored.	Yes	No
7.	I often felt guilty.	Yes	No
8.	I often felt I was being punished.	Yes	No
9.	I often felt disappointed in myself.	Yes	No
10.	I often hated myself.	Yes	No

11.	I blamed myself for bad things that happened.	Yes	No
12.	I cried a lot.	Yes	No
13.	I often felt irritable.	Yes	No
14.	I didn't care about what was happening around me.	Yes	No
15.	I didn't care about other people.	Yes	No
16.	I couldn't make decisions.	Yes	No
17.	I often felt unattractive.	Yes	No
18.	I couldn't work.	Yes	No
19.	I couldn't fall asleep.	Yes	No
20.	I couldn't stay awake.	Yes	No
21.	I often felt tired.	Yes	No
22.	I often had no appetite.	Yes	No
23.	I didn't care about sex.	Yes	No
24.	I worried about everything.	Yes	No
25.	I often felt ashamed.	Yes	No

If you answered "Yes" to ten or more questions you are probably depressed. If you answered "Yes" to fifteen or more questions you are depressed. Discuss this with your spouse, family, minister, and doctor. If you thought of ending your life, seek help immediately!

Physical Symptoms of Depression

Depressed people, like anxious people, can have physical symptoms. Many anxiety-related physical symptoms result from an overactive sympathetic nervous system. Part of the calming response is to turn down the sympathetic nervous system and turn on the parasympathetic nervous system. Many depression-related symptoms may result from a sympathetic nervous system that is turned down too much, or a parasympathetic nervous system that is turned up too much. The symptoms of depression may be different from those of anxiety.

1. *Depressed person:* I often feel my hands or feet are cold, numb, or painful.
   Anxious person: I often feel my hands or feet are tingling or burning.

2. *Depressed person:* I often feel cold or blue.
   Anxious person: I often feel flushed.
3. *Depressed person:* I often feel awful, miserable, or in pain.
   Anxious person: I feel unsteady or wobbly.
4. *Depressed person:* I often feel everything's black before my eyes.
   Anxious person: I often feel my vision is blurred.
5. *Depressed person:* I often feel awful, or miserable, or in pain.
   Anxious person: I often feel dizzy or lightheaded.
6. *Depressed person:* I often feel I can't move, or I'm paralyzed.
   Anxious person: I often feel I'm shaking or trembling.
7. *Depressed person:* I often feel I can't move, or I'm paralyzed.
   Anxious person: I often feel I'm restless or jumpy.
8. *Depressed person:* I often feel I'm suffocating, or I can't breath, or I'm dying.
   Anxious person: I feel short of breath.
9. *Depressed person:* I often feel awful, miserable, or in pain.
   Anxious person: I often feel nauseated.
10. *Depressed person:* I often feel cold or frozen.
    Anxious person: I often feel hot or cold flashes.

The range of responses is greater among anxious people. If you're anxious you may have at least one symptom for each question. If you're depressed you may answer "I often feel awful, or miserable, or in pain," or "I often feel I can't move or I'm paralyzed" over and over. A restricted range of responses is part of being depressed.

How Many People Are Depressed?

Of the 27 million Americans who are anxious, about 4.5 million are depressed. In some, depression precedes anxiety, in others it follows anxiety, and in many depression and anxiety occur together and is called anxious or agitated depression (Figure 8.1). In addition, 4.5 million people are depressed without being anxious. In about half of depressed people, the depression occurs in reaction to an external situation. This is called a reactive, situational, or external depression, which can result from the loss of a parent, a spouse, another family member, a friend, a favorite animal, or a famous person whom you admired, such as President Kennedy, Dr. Martin Luther King Jr., or Princess Diana. This can also result from the loss of a job or the break up of a marriage or relationship.

Depression can, as it did in Anna from Chapter 1, result from being diagnosed with PD and reading about the disease. This depression, one resulting from bad information, can be corrected by good information. Depression can, as it did in Jack Jr. from Chapter 2, result from being diagnosed with PD and believing your PD will follow the same path as your father's. This depression can be corrected by good advice. Depression can result from anxiety. This could happen to Martha from Chapter 7.

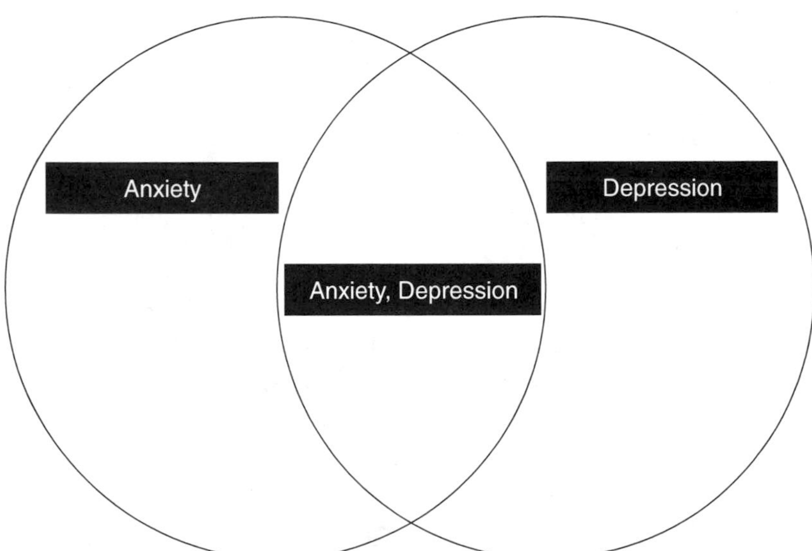

Figure 8.1 *In Some People, Anxiety and Depression Occur, Creating a State Called Agitated (Anxious) Depression*

Parkinson disease, even when it's advanced, need not be accompanied by depression. Listen to Norma Udall, a prominent Washington lobbyist, speaking about her husband, Congressman Morris Udall.

When I married Mo, I knew he had PD. Mo, a great speaker, had lost his ability to speak. And being unable to show expression with his face made it difficult to know what he was thinking. Parkinson impacted our lives and our marriage every day. But because we'd known each other for many years, we spoke without talking. And we continued doing things together. Try to make life as easy as you can for your partner, but don't take away their dignity.

Dan, a 60-Year-Old Man Who Is Depressed

I was 60 years old when I was diagnosed with Parkinson. I'm a banker, we had merged, and I was forced out. I received a generous settlement and could comfortably retire. But I was angry, resentful, and depressed. I looked depressed: I didn't smile, my face was masked, expressionless. I walked stooped-over as though I was carrying the world on my shoulders. And I moved slowly because, I thought, I'm retired and I'm 60 — six, O — the male menopause. I didn't think I got on people's nerves, but I did. And Barbara, my wife, insisted I see a "shrink." The "shrink" stunned me. He said I was depressed, of course, but he also said, "and you have PD."

"Parkinson disease!" I gasped. " My father-in-law had PD. And my brother-in-law has PD. So I can't have PD."

A specialist confirmed the diagnosis. "Forty percent of PD people are depressed," he said, "In some, like you, the depression's reactive, related to outside events: losing your job, turning 60. And in some, it's part of the disease. And, as the outer features of depression and PD are similar: masked face, stooped posture, slowed movement, one can be overlooked in the presence of the other."

That's what happened with me. I missed it and so did Barbara. My father-in-law, Jack Sr., had PD, and when his wife died, he moved in with us. Barbara became his care partner. It was the right thing to do but I resented it. And of course you can't tell your wife you're resentful because she's spending more time with her father than you. After Jack Sr. died, and I thought I had Barbara to myself, her brother, Jack Jr., developed PD.

Because Jack's father had PD he was a basket case. And Barbara became his care partner. Now I was a basket case.

Barbara's a saint. She has enough understanding for a dozen basket cases, but I'm no saint — I was angry and upset. I'm not religious, I don't believe in God, but I was convinced God was punishing me for resenting Barbara's attention to her father. It's not logical or rational but it's how my mind works. The shrink started me on Zoloft. And the PD specialist started me on Sinemet and, then Sinemet with Comtan. And, although I improved physically and psychologically I still couldn't do everything I should do because I remained angry and upset. I was a Stage 2 Parkinson but I acted like a Stage 5.

Barbara's a rock, my support, and so's the shrink — but it takes time to work out your feelings. I'm still angry and upset at the bank, and at Jack Jr., but, as time passes, the anger is less. I have difficulty sleeping. In part because I have PD and I can't turn in bed. And in part because I wake up imagining I'm fighting with my father-in-law and brother-in-law screaming at them for taking Barbara away from me. The Zoloft is beginning to help. It's not a happiness pill but I'm less anxious, less upset. It's a question of coming to terms with myself. "It's no different," says Barbara, who goes to church regularly and reads the Bible, "from Job working out his anger against God."

From the Book of Job

In my anguish of spirit I speak, in my bitterness of soul I complain.

If I say my bed will comfort me, my couch will lighten my complaints.

You frighten me with dreams and terrify me with visions.

I am wasting away, my life is unending.

If I have sinned, what is it I have done

That You choose me as Your target?

My Mobility Index is 16 (out of 40). Everything's an ordeal.

My Emotional Index is 31 (out of 44).

My Autonomic Index is 10 (out of 16).

My score on the Quality of Life Scale is 57%.

I consider my quality of life as bad — but improving.

What Depression Does to a Person with Parkinson Disease

Depression occurs in about 40% of people with PD. It's usually an integral part of PD, unrelated to the degree or duration of symptoms. In 20% of people with PD who are depressed, the depression precedes the onset of PD, something appreciated only after you've been diagnosed with PD (this is what happened in Dan). In addition to an internal, or endogenous, depression PD people may suffer from a situational depression, one related to an event such as retirement (as happened in Dan), or knowledge of a relative with PD (as happened in Jack Jr.) (Figure 8.2). In some PD people the depression is associated with anxiety and in them the anxiety may be overwhelming, resulting in an agitated depression. In some people PD is complicated by autonomic nervous system symptoms, in some by difficulty sleeping, in some by an intellectual decline. Depression can make everything worse.

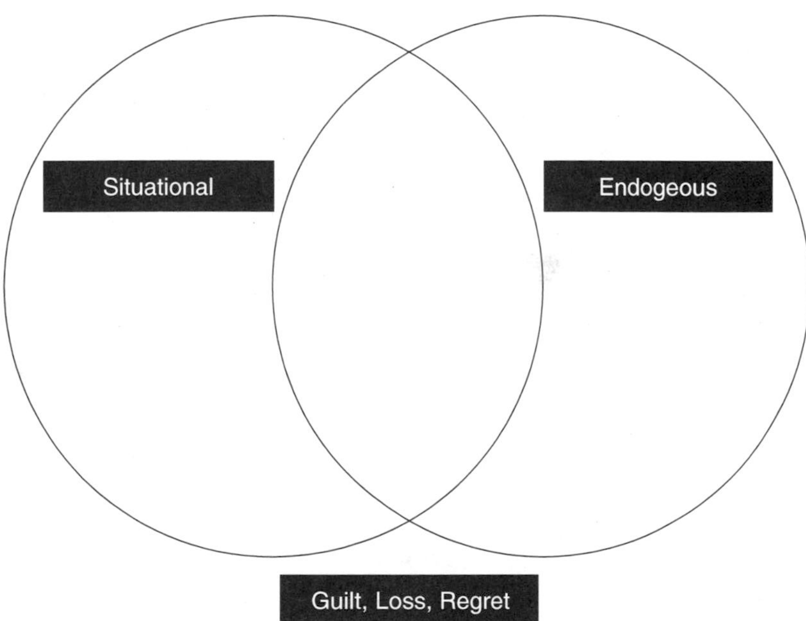

Figure 8.2 *Situational and Endogenous Depression Can Contribute to Feelings of Guilt, Loss, and Regret.*

The Apathetic Depression

Perhaps 25% of PD people suffer from apathy, drowsiness, fatigue, no energy, and passivity. This is called an apathetic depression although many people deny they're depressed. The apathetic depression of PD may be different from other kinds of depression, may be accompanied by an intellectual decline, and may not respond to antidepression drugs.

The Anatomy of Depression

The symptoms of PD result from a loss of dopamine nerve cells in the substantia nigra. Accompanying this is a loss of norepinephrine nerve cells in a nearby region, the locus ceruleus. Norepinephrine is a naturally occurring chemical involved in regulating the autonomic nervous system. A lack of brain norepinephrine may be responsible, in part, for depression.

Treating Depression

Many of the ways of reducing anxiety can reduce depression. If you are depressed, meditation, counseling, exercise, and breathing techniques as discussed in Chapter 7 may help you. Improving your PD can also reduce depression. The selective serotonin re-uptake inhibitors, the SSRIs, are effective in depression. The doses of the SSRIs are similar for depression and anxiety. The dose must be discussed with your doctor. If you are taking selegiline, caution is advised if you need an SSRI. Inside the brain, the increased serotonin released by the SSRIs is broken down by an enzyme, MAO-A. Selegiline at the doses used in PD, 5 to 10 mg a day, block an enzyme, MAO-B, a cousin of MAO-A. If you are taking more than 10 mg of selegiline a day, the extra selegiline blocks MAO-A. This can result in increased concentrations of serotonin resulting in side effects such as agitation, confusion, hallucinations, fever, flushing, shivering, and sweating. As a rule, selegiline is usually stopped before starting an SSRI. The two most widely used SSRIs for the anxious depression of PD are Paxil and Zoloft. The most widely used SSRI for the apathetic depression of PD is Prozac. The following drugs are also used in treating the depression of PD. When, why, and how they are prescribed is at the discretion of your doctor.

Effexor (Venlafaxine) increases brain norepinephrine and serotonin. It may be helpful when an SSRI isn't. Its half-life is 5 hours. The dose is 25 to 75 mg, two to three times a day.

Wellbutrin (bupropion) increases brain dopamine levels in all regions of the brain, not just the ones impacted by PD. It is helpful in the apathetic depression of PD. Side effects include agitation, confusion, delusions, and hallucinations, these are more likely in older people.

Tricyclic antidepressants (TCAs) consist of a molecule made up of three rings joined together. TCAs block the reuptake of norepinephrine and serotonin, increasing their concentration in specific brain regions. The TCAs were the first antidepressants but have been replaced by SSRIs. TCAs differ in their side effects, including their ability to cause drowsiness. This is an advantage if you are depressed and having difficulty sleeping, and a disadvantage if you must stay alert. The TCAs partially block the parasympathetic nervous system. This may result in side effects such as dry mouth, a fast heart rate, constipation, an irritable bladder, and impotence. Agitation, confusion, delusions, and hallucinations can occur in older or intellectually impaired people. The TCAs are stopped because of side effects in less than 5% of people. The TCAs are helpful in a variety of pain syndromes. In part, TCAs decrease pain by decreasing the anxiety and depression that accompany pain. However, SSRIs are more effective in decreasing anxiety and depression but aren't as effective in decreasing pain. This suggests that TCAs may decrease pain, in part, by blocking the parasympathetic nervous system that may contribute to pain. TCAs include:

- *Elavil (Amitriptyline)*. It peaks in 2 to 4 hours. Its half-life is 10 to 50 hours. The dose is 25 to 200 mg a day. It is used for depression, difficulty sleeping, panic, and pain.
- *Pamelor (Nortriptyline)* is the chief metabolite of Elavil. It is faster acting than Elavil and has similar uses. The dose is 50 to 150 mg a day.
- *Sinequan (Doxepin)*. Its half-life is 8 to 24 hours. It is used for depression, difficulty sleeping and panic. The dose is 50 to 200 mg a day.
- *Tofranil (Impramine)*. It peaks in 2 to 4 hours. Its half-life is 6 to 20 hours. It is used for anxiety, depression, enuresis (bed-wetting), and panic. The dose is 25 to 200 mg a day.

Monoamine Oxidase-A (MAO-A) Inhibitors. Nardil (Phenelzine) and Parnate (Tranylcypromine) block an enzyme, MAO-A that breaks down dopamine, norepinephrine, and serotonin. Blocking MAO-A increases the concentration of these naturally occurring brain chemicals. MAO inhibitors are slow acting but may be effective in depressions not responding to SSRIs, TCAs, or other drugs. MAO-A inhibitors must not be combined with SSRIs or TCAs as the combination can markedly increase norepinephrine and serotonin, which may result in dangerously high blood pressure. People taking MAO inhibitors cannot eat foods that contain tyramine, an norepinephrine-like chemical. Eating these foods, such as aged cheeses and red wines, while taking an MAO inhibitor can also result in high blood pressure. Depression in PD is not permanent, so PD people may not have to take antidepression drugs for life.

Electric Shock. If meditation, counseling, and drugs fail, electroconvulsive shock therapy (ECT) can help selected people. ECT is no longer the horror portrayed in Ken Kesey's *One Flew Over the Cuckoo's Nest.* ECT is done under sedation using muscle relaxants to confine the seizure to the brain, not the body. In some people there's a temporary loss of memory. And, in some people there's a temporary reduction in PD symptoms. Newer techniques, now under study, include stimulation of the vagus nerve (the main outflow of the parasympathetic nervous system), deep brain stimulation (DBS) of regions near the locus ceruleus, and transmagnetic cranial stimulation, a technique that results in milder seizures than those caused by electricity.

In dealing with depression, remember the Bible. If God is all caring, why is there PD? Is it a part of a Divine Plan to unlock the brain's secrets? Look to the Book of Job.

GOD MOVES THE MOUNTAINS, THOUGH THEY DO NOT KNOW IT.
GOD THROWS THEM DOWN WHEN HE IS ANGRY,
GOD SHAKES THE EARTH, AND MOVES IT FROM ITS PLACE,
MAKING ALL ITS PILLARS TREMBLE.
THE SUN, AT GOD'S COMMAND, WILL NOT RISE,
AND ON THE STARS GOD SETS A SEAL.
GOD AND NO OTHER HAS STRETCHED OUT THE HEAVENS.
AND TRAMPLED DOWN THE WAVES OF THE SEA.
GOD'S WORKS ARE GREAT AND UNFATHOMABLE,
AND GOD'S MARVELS CANNOT BE COUNTED.
IF GOD PASSES ME, I DO NOT SEE GOD
NOR DO I KNOW HIS MIND.

And from Isaiah

FOR I WILL CREATE NEW HEAVENS AND A NEW EARTH.
THE PAST WILL BE NOT BE REMEMBERED,
AND WILL COME NO MORE TO MIND.
NO MORE WILL THE SOUND OF WEEPING BE HEARD,
NOR THE SOUND OF SHRIEKING.

People will build houses and live in them,
They will plant vineyards and eat their fruit.
They will not toil in vain.
Before they call, I shall answer.
Before they speak, I shall have heard.

Care Partners, the First Defense

If you develop PD, everyone in your family is affected, and everyone's role changes. Having a network of people makes a difference. If you find it difficult to rely on others, you must change. Remember, as well as getting help, you will be able to help. Helping others, giving of yourself, is an antidote for loneliness. Jack Jr. from Chapter 2 got help from Lenny. And Lenny enjoyed helping Jack. Jerry, the dentist, got help from Martha. And Martha, in helping Jerry, came to terms with her PD.

As PD advances, you and your partner will change. Who are the caregivers, these messengers from God? In 1997, the National Family Caregivers Association polled its members, people who care for children, spouses, and parents with chronic diseases, and found:

- 80% of care partners are women
- 50% care for a spouse, 25% care for a parent
- 70% are between the ages 36 and 65
- 60% spend at least 40 hours a week caregiving
- 50% of caregivers also work outside the home
- 70% of caregivers work at least 30 hours a week

Although men and women become ill equally, 80% of caregivers are women. Why? Caregiving has been and still is traditionally a woman's role. Although their roles are changing, women maintain their strong maternal instincts. Although it is common for women to work outside the home, the majority of people with PD come from a time when women didn't do men's work and vice versa. For most men with PD, women are natural caregivers. Lenny readily accepted Laurie's help, and Jack Jr. readily accepted his sister, Barbara's help. In contrast, Anna went through a transition, first accepting help from her daughter, Nancy, then from her husband Bruce.

Caregivers — Be Flexible

Think back to when you were in charge of a big project. First you identified what had to be done, then how to do it, and finally who could do it. You weighed everyone's abilities, talents, and availability. Then you assigned roles. The same process must be used to create a plan to cope with PD. The two key people are you and your partner. "The most important thing is being flexible," says Laurie. "Facing PD is like riding a roller coaster — once you've hurtled around one curve, and things have settled down, a new and more dangerous curve appears. You must adjust. When I was diagnosed with Hodgkin's disease, Lenny rode the roller coaster with me. Could I do less for him?"

Often people approach situations with fixed ideas. For example, in many homes a woman is responsible for raising the children and keeping the house, even if she has a full-time career. A man is responsible for finances. Melvin, the state senator, and Jane, his wife, are a typical household. When Mel was diagnosed with PD, he was at the peak of his career. Mel's staff didn't want him to admit he had PD, they were afraid he wouldn't be re-elected. Jane wanted Mel to admit he had PD, it would be easier, less stressful on him. Mel, while agreeing with Jane, followed his staff's advice: in his heart he had not accepted that he had PD, and he wasn't ready to change roles. But in time, as Mel adjusted to PD, he accepted his limitations, and he admitted his reliance on Jane. When Mel decided not to run for governor, Jane was the obvious choice. In working with Mel, Jane had shown her judgment and reliability. For Mel, letting Jane take his place was a sign, not of weakness, but of strength — and wisdom.

Care Partners — Don't Burn Out

Being a care partner is a full-time job. Respect each other, don't burn each other out. The following are suggestions from successful care partners, Anna and Bruce, Mel and Jane, Lenny and Laurie.

1. Allow more time for everything. Be patient.
2. Know each other; ask each other what you can or can't do.
3. Allow PD people to do as much for themselves as possible. If you think they need help, ask. If they say no, let them do for themselves. If they can't, don't say, "I told you I should help." Instead say, "let's try it again — together." Doing it together maintains their pride.

Some PD people lose their ability to realize they can't do certain things like drive a car. It is not denial, a conscious blotting out of information; it is a subconscious blotting out of information. It is related to why PD people have symptoms, aren't aware of their symptoms, and aren't diagnosed — for years. PD affects automatic activities, activities that run on autopilot. Just as you may not be aware that your plane is operating on autopilot, so the PD person may not be aware he's operating on autopilot.

Care partners must look out for each other; the caregiver for the person with PD and vice versa. If you are the person with PD, each day, just as your spouse asks you how you're doing, ask her how she's doing. She may be as tired from caring as you are from PD. And she's as much in need of a hug from you as you are from her.

Caregivers — Learn as Much as You Can

If your spouse has PD, learn as much as you can. But beware of misinformation and of drawing false conclusions. A case in point is Bruce, Anna's husband. Bruce went to a care partner's support group for the first time. There he overheard people talking about a drug their spouses with PD were taking. They raved about a magical gel-filled capsule and how it really did the trick. Too afraid to speak up and ask how the drug helped their spouses, Bruce jotted down the drug's name and left the meeting. All night he wondered why Anna's doctor hadn't prescribed this "magical" drug for Anna. Almost everyone else was taking it. Bruce began to doubt the doctor's choice of treatment and his expertise! Finally, Bruce called the doctor's office and asked why Anna wasn't getting what he had decided was the best drug for PD. The doctor cleared Bruce's confusion with a short explanation, "that drug is for constipation, and Anna isn't constipated."

Caregivers — Prepare

1. **Learn what resources are available.** Find a medical facility nearby that provides medical and rehabilitative services specifically for PD. Develop a relationship with members of your spouse's treatment team, including the primary care doctor (people with PD get other diseases as well as PD), the neurologist, the nurse, the pharmacist, the physical therapist, and the social worker.
2. **Think about an emergency.** If you can't be reached and there's an emergency at home, who will call the doctor or ambulance? Or, if your spouse needs care and you're not available, whom can you call to take your place? All problems can be solved with planning.

   Make a list of important phone numbers and leave the list by the phone. Prepare a binder of vital information, duplicate it, carry one copy with you, and leave the other in a prominent place at home.
3. **Make your home safe.** People with PD have trouble walking in cluttered spaces. Widen the areas in which your spouse walks, and get rid of objects he can trip over. Install guard rails in the bathroom and shower, and make sure your stairway railings are secure. Clear an empty space in the middle of one room so your spouse can walk in an open space. An occupational or a physical therapist can come to your home and give you advice.
4. **Learn about medical equipment — even if it is not needed.** Learn about any device that can help your spouse do difficult tasks such as buttoning a shirt button, lacing shoes, and other activities of daily living. Learn about walkers, canes, and walking sticks. Canes are easy to use, but they're often too low and

force a person to bend, making them take extra steps. To experience this, try walking while bending from the waist. Walking sticks may be harder to use, but by helping a person to walk upright, walking sticks result in a person taking a longer, more natural stride. Remember Moses used a walking stick to navigate the Sinai. And it took 40 years. If Moses had used a cane — he'd never have crossed the Red Sea. More than reading, the devices teach you about walking.

5. **Learn good ways of caregiving.** Learn how to lift, transfer, and bathe. Ask a nurse or physical therapist to teach you how to do each of these techniques. Learning how to do them properly and efficiently will make your job less tiring. Learn from the American Red Cross how to take a blood pressure, a pulse rate, a breathing rate. It's no more difficult than using a thermometer. And learn about CPR. Boy scouts do it, girl scouts do it, you can do it.
6. **Learn about finances and legalities.** Is your spouse working? If so, how long will he be able to work? Does he have disability insurance, or private health insurance, Medicare, or long-term care insurance? Does he have a Living Will or a Last Will and Testament? You'll need to learn about his estate, because it's also your estate. And get a durable power of attorney so you can do things when your spouse can't.
7. **Learn about support groups.** Are there support groups for your partner? For you? You may feel alone, but you're not. Lenny and Laurie started a support group. Jerry, the dentist, Jack Jr., and Dan all benefited by going to it. And who but a PD support group can listen and give advice on the every day problems of PD — like a PD support group?

Caregivers — Care for Yourself

Caregiving is rewarding — but exhausting. Are you taking care of yourself? Your health may seem unimportant compared to your spouse's PD, but if you become sick, who will care for your spouse? Exercise, get enough sleep, and take time to relax. In 1997, the National Family Caregivers Association survey revealed good and bad aspects of caregiving:

- 70% of caregivers found an "inner strength" they never knew they had.
- 35% became closer to their spouse.
- 67% were frustrated.
- 60% were depressed.

A study by Julie Carter, RN, of the NPF Center of Excellence in Oregon of 380 caregivers showed a link between caregiver strain and advancing PD.

- In Stage 1 PD, caregivers performed 11 of 51 tasks, 21% of tasks for their spouses.
- In Stage 2 PD, caregivers performed 18 of 51 tasks, 35% of tasks for their spouses.
- In Stage 3 PD, caregivers performed 24 of 51 tasks, 47% of tasks for their spouses.
- In Stage 4 PD, caregivers performed 30 of 51 tasks, 58% of tasks for their spouses.

As PD advances, caregivers must perform more and more tasks for their spouses; the more tasks they perform, the more physically and mentally strained they become.

As PD advances, as you take on more tasks, you will feel strained. Take the Anxiety Questionnaire. Take the Depression Questionnaire. If you are anxious or depressed — seek treatment. Anxiety and depression in you can be as bad as in your spouse.

Treating Caregiver Strain

Look to meditation, exercise, breathing techniques, counseling, and, if necessary, medication if you are feeling strained. Take time for yourself — without feeling guilty. If you crack, who will look after your partner? A week or two off can revitalize you — and your spouse; plan carefully.

Determine how many hours per week you devote to caregiving. If the total exceeds 40 hours per week, you need more help — and rest.

Get your families to help. Dan's wife, Barbara, was a caregiver to her father, her brother, but she was neglecting Dan — and he became depressed. Why doesn't Jack Jr.'s wife, help? How long can Barbara continue to be "Wonder Woman"? Not long, if Dan cracks.

"Care-pool." Through your support group, you'll find other caregivers who need a break. Care-pool — you care for one person's partner while caring for your own (at your home) once a week. Then that person can care for both at their home once a week. You'll have a few hours to yourself and so will the other caregiver. This is what Barbara and Jack Jr.'s wife did.

Stay connected with your family, friends, community, and yourself. If you celebrated Thanksgiving or Christmas at your home with your family, continue doing so. But don't do everything yourself. Call, visit, write, e-mail, or go out with your friends regularly. If you've been active in community affairs, continue — in the enjoyable ones. Keep up your interests, your hobbies, and exercise. Don't be a one-dimensional person: caregiving, caregiving, caregiving — it's not good for you or your partner. Two or more other activities make you a three-dimensional person: a better person, caregiver, and partner. Maintain a sense of humor, laugh at yourself: laughter is the best medicine.

Jill, the wife of Jack Jr., and the daughter-in-law of Jack Sr., was not, in the beginning, a sympathetic care partner. She was criticized by family, friends, and by Jack Sr.'s and Jack Jr.'s doctors, for not being more caring. To which she replied, "Don't rush to judgment. There are things I know that you don't."

Jill, a 55-Year-Old Woman Who Does Not Have Parkinson Disease

My name is Jill, I'm a doctor, a "shrink." I've written popular books, bestsellers, on aging, sadness, and depression: Old Age is a Downer *and*

Growing Old is Bad For Your Health. *I've also written, serious, scholarly books:* The Dynamics of Depression, *and the* Geriatrician's Bible. *I'm a professor of psychiatry at the university, I'm on the book and lecture circuit, and I have my own radio call-in show.*

You know my husband, Jack Jr., the lawyer with PD who discovered it in himself by studying his handwriting. And you know Jack's father, Jack Sr., who had PD. And you know how Jack Jr. "freaked out" when he discovered he had PD. And you must know I wasn't Jack Jr.'s rock, his support. Barbara, my sister-in-law, cared for Jack Sr., and now she's caring for her husband, Dan, who has PD and is depressed, and she's also caring for Jack Jr. because I can't. It sounds like, and perhaps it is, The Days of Our Lives *in Parkinson Disease. Barbara is a saint, Saint Barbara. And if I were as mean-spirited as some people think, I'd resent Barbara for being so caring. But I don't. Can you hate Mother Theresa?*

Another thing, I'm Jill, and my husband's Jack — and it's not a nursery rhyme. I'm Jewish, at least that's what I put down when I'm asked where I'd like to be buried. My father, Jakob, was religious and so was my mother, and a lot of good it did. My parents survived the holocaust. Jakob, a master tailor, made uniforms for the Nazi "big wigs." Imagine, the Nazi "big wigs" dressed in clothes made by a Jew. And my mother, Rachel, survived by working as a cleaning girl. If a man's naked, and he's a Jew, you know he's a naked Jew. But if a woman's naked, she's a naked woman. When the War ended, and concentration camps were emptied, Jakob met Jack Sr., a colonel in Army intelligence. They became friends, and after the war, Jack Sr. brought my parents, and now me, to America.

Jakob opened a custom tailor shop in town — and prospered. Rachel, worn out from the War, died. They said she ruptured an aneurysm in her brain. It wasn't an aneurysm, it was her soul. Jakob believed in God, said God saved us, and read the Bible, the Old Testament, every day. I thought that it was nonsense: filled with contradictions, fairy tales, and lust. First God creates the earth, then like a child tiring of a toy, he drowns everyone except Noah. Then, like a roller-coaster, when you think everything's okay God strikes again — He destroys Sodom and Gomorra. Of course He saves Lot, and his daughters, but He turns Lot's wife into a pillar of salt, because she dared to gaze at the havoc God wrought. It's more than Lot's wife. Read the story of Judah, the brother of Joseph, the sons of Jakob.

From the Book of Genesis.

"And it came to pass that Judah wed a Canaanite woman whose name was Shua and Shua bore a son whose name was Er. And Shua conceived again and bore a son whose name was Onan. And she yet again bore Shua a son whose name was Shelah. And Judah took a wife for Er, and her name was Tamar. Er was wicked in the sight of God, and God slew him. And Judah said onto Onan, as was the custom,

"Go in unto thy brother's wife, Tamar, and perform the duty of a husband. And raise up seed to thy brother."

And it came to pass, when Onan went in unto his brother's wife, he spilled his seed on the ground, lest he should give seed to his brother's wife. And the thing which he did displeased God and God slew Onan.

Then said Judah to Tamar, his daughter-in-law, "remain a widow in my house, till Shelah my son is grown." And Tamar went and dwelt in Judah's house. And in time, Judah's wife died. And in time, Tamar put off the garments of her widowhood and covered herself with her veil, and wrapped herself and sat where Judah saw her and thought her to be a harlot for she had covered her face.

Judah turned her way and because he knew not she was his daughter-in-law, said, "Come I pray thee let me come unto thee."

And Tamar said, "What will you give me, that thou may come in unto me?" And Judah said, "What shall I give thee?"

And Tamar said, "Give me thy signet and thy cord, and thy staff that is in thy hand."

And Judah gave them to her, and came in unto her."

Maybe Judah knew he was speaking to Tamar and maybe he didn't. A biblical scholar, Jonathan Kirsch wrote, "We might imagine that Judah actually recognizes Tamar, behind the veil and that he has longed for her even when she was married to his sons, that he seizes the chance to act on his longing. Perhaps the harlot's disguise is a game that each of them plays by prior arrangement to titillate each other, or to provide a plausible denial."

And Tamar arose and went away and put off her veil from her, and put on the garments of her widowhood and it came to pass about three months after, that it was told Judah that Tamar his daughter-in-law had played the harlot and moreover she was with child. Judah acknowledged them, and said, "You are more righteous than I."

Jack Sr., was a father to me more than my father, Jakob. And when Jakob died, Jack Sr. paid for college and medical school. And it wasn't about my being a father to a daughter. Jack Sr. and I were lovers, and I married Jack Jr., because I couldn't marry Jack Sr. So when Jack Sr. developed PD I felt, in a deep, troubled, and improbable way, that God had punished Jack Sr. because of me. And I was to blame for his PD. Perhaps, then you'll understand why I could not be Jack Sr.'s care partner. After Jack Sr. died, Jack Jr., my husband, developed PD and again I ran away. I am a psychiatrist, I do understand how I feel, and I've begun to come to terms with myself — and God. God created the earth, but he gave us free will, and we abuse it. Although Tamar may have lured Judah, God didn't force Judah on her. And although I may have lured Jack Sr., God didn't force him on me. I guess what I'm saying is when a man rejects his wife because she develops PD, or vice versa, it may not be PD. It's probably something neither of them has told the other, or their doctor.

If you are a caregiver, and caregiving is difficult, look to God. Read the Bible. The Bible is like life, a sea of happenings, with good and bad. And there are contradictions in the Bible. But the Bible is, like life, a repository of wisdom. Anyone can believe when things go well. But, when things go badly, it's even more important to believe.

In describing God, the Book of Psalms is describing caregivers.

YOU ARE LIKE A SHELTER FROM THE WIND, A REFUGE FROM THE STORM.
YOU ARE LIKE A STREAM ON ARID GROUND,
LIKE THE SHADE OF A ROCK IN A DESOLATE LAND.
THROUGH YOU MY EYES WILL NO LONGER BE CLOSED,
MY EARS WILL REMAIN UNSTOPPED.
MY HEART WILL LEARN TO CONSIDER,
AND MY STUTTERING TONGUE WILL SPEAK CLEARLY.

CHAPTER

9

Parkinson and Dementia

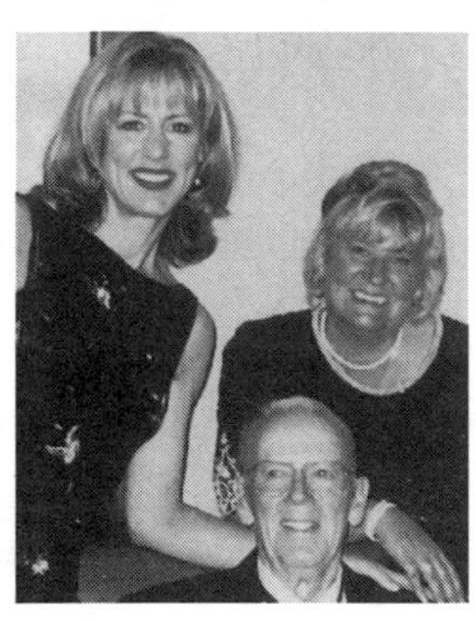

Christine Lahti, Actress, shown here with her sister and father

"You should understand how to help your parent if he or she has Parkinson disease. You need to know that they have to keep exercising and stay independent as long as possible. The tendency I think is to become very dependent and scared, but the longer they can stay active and strong, the better their quality of life will be.

"Since this interview was given, I am terribly saddened to report that my dad's Parkinson has progressed rapidly. It's incredibly painful to see a parent become so helpless because of Parkinson disease.

"Miraculously, he still has his sense of humor — he can still laugh at his favorite jokes and can even sing a few bars from his favorite songs. I know he still recognizes me and my brothers and sisters but that ability too, seems to be fading.

"Very few people, I find, ever talk about the final stages of this devastating disease. But maybe that's one of the reasons we don't have a cure yet — because not enough people really recognize the urgent need for one. I know my Dad would want the truth to be told if, in any way, his story could help toward finding that cure.

"Although it's too late for him, there's every reason for many of you reading this book to have tremendous hope. Given the recent breakthroughs in research, there's good reason to believe a cure will be found. But is must be found *soon.*"

What is Dementia?

Dementia is an overall or global decline in intellect and is the most feared complication of PD. The outward features of dementia are obvious: confusion, memory loss, unusual behavior, and daytime drowsiness. Of the one million people with PD now living, 30%, or 300,000, have or will develop dementia. People with PD age 70 years or older are at greater risk for dementia. Of the 20% or 200,000 people with PD who eventually need care outside the home including a nursing home, 80% of the 20%, or 160,000 people, need care because of dementia. The economic cost of caring for a PD person with dementia is 10 times the cost of caring for a PD person without dementia. The emotional and spiritual cost of caring for a PD person with dementia cannot be measured.

Dementia results from a loss of cells throughout the brain, not a loss confined to a specific region. The number of lost cells needed to cause dementia will vary depending upon the regions of the brain affected, and the disease causing the dementia. Among the diseases causing dementia are Alzheimer, PD, Diffuse Lewy Body Disease, brain injury, infection, and stroke. And the dementia of each is different. Although the figures are inexact, the person with dementia suffers a 30 to 70% loss of IQ.

Dementia Is Different from Psychosis and Coma

Dementia may be preceded, accompanied, or followed by psychosis. Or dementia and psychosis may appear separately. Psychosis is a blend of hallucinations, delusions, agitation, rage, and mood swings. Just as several diseases can cause dementia, several conditions can cause psychosis, including brain injuries, drugs, (legal and illegal), and schizophrenia. Dementia is permanent and progressive. Psychosis is usually temporary. The person with dementia or psychosis is awake and can be talked to although he may not understand or listen. The person in a coma is not awake and cannot listen. Think of the brain as a computer. Dementia affects the hardware: the hard drive, the chips, and the wiring. Psychosis affects the software, the programming. And coma affects the power source.

Intellectual Decline Is Not Dementia

The dementia of PD may be preceded by a stage of intellectual decline. This decline is subtle and may not be appreciated by the person with PD. It may show up as difficulty in balancing the checkbook, difficulty in using a computer, difficulty in driving or parking the car, or excessive daytime drowsiness. Some doctors refer to it as bradyphrenia, slowness of thinking similar to bradykinesia (slowness of moving). At the level of the brain, as distinct from the soul, moving and thinking are similar, both require the coordination and firing of multiple brain cells. A disease like PD that can slow movement can also slow thinking. A note of caution: such slow thinking may also be a feature of depression. Identifying the intellectual decline, sorting it out from depression, and starting drugs to prevent it from progressing to dementia are important future developments.

How Is Dementia Diagnosed? The Mini-Mental Status Examination (MMSE)

To diagnose dementia and follow its course, doctors do a Mini-Mental Status Examination. There are more detailed examinations than the MMSE but they are not as widely used or accepted. The MMSE consists of a series of questions. These include:

1. **Questions on orientation and general information.** The person with PD is asked to name the day of the week, the day of the month, the month, the year, the name of the county, city, and state in which the person lives. (Total 7 points)

   The person is asked to name the president and vice president of the United States, and the governor of the state in which he lives. (Total 3 points)
2. **Questions on short-term memory and attention span.** The person is given three paired objects to remember. After the objects are named, the person is asked to repeat them. He must remember both objects of each pair. Typical paired objects are red hen, black goose, or 300 dollars. (Total 3 points)

   The person is then asked to spell the word *world* backwards. (Total 5 points, one for each correct letter)

   The person is again given three paired objects; the same three paired objects as before. He must remember both objects of each pair. (Total 3 points)
3. **Questions on language, ability to tell left from right, reading, and writing.** The person is asked to repeat a phrase such as: "No ifs, ands, or buts about it."

   The person is asked to follow a command such as: "Take your right hand, place it on your head, and comb your hair." The person is asked to name objects such as a hand, a thumb, and an ear. The person is asked to read the phrase: "close your eyes." The person is asked to write the phrase: "close your eyes." The person is asked to obey the command: "close your eyes." (Total 8 points)
4. **Questions on visual spatial orientation.** The person is asked to copy a diagram. The person is asked to complete a design. (Total 2 points)

The total available points is 30 points. A MMSE score of 27–30 is normal; a MMSE score of 24–26 is borderline, the person may have dementia. A MMSE score of 23 or less is abnormal, the person has dementia. In people with Alzheimer disease, each year the MMSE score declines by three points.

The difficulty with using the MMSE in people with PD is that it was designed for people with Alzheimer disease, which is different from the dementia of PD. In Alzheimer disease the ability to use words to describe things is heavily impacted, whereas in PD it is not. The person with PD may have difficulty speaking loudly or distinctly but not in describing things. Because of this, I use a different scale. Unlike the MMSE, it hasn't been validated but it brings forth, often to the surprise of the person with PD and his family, the extent of the problem.

The Parkinson Mini-Mental Status Examination (PMMSE)

Questions on Orientation and General Information

The person is asked the month, the year, the name of the president, and the doctor's name. I don't ask people to tell me the name of the vice president, or the name of the governor of their state. Many normal people do not know the name of the vice president, nor do they know the name of the governor of their state. They will ask, "Is it the governor of the state we live in during the summer? Or the governor of the state we live in during the winter?" The person is also asked about a recent event, one's that's been widely reported in the news. These questions test the whole brain. *Total 5 points.*

Questions on Short-Term Memory and Attention Span

This is the same as in the MMSE, except spelling *world* backwards scores 1 not 5 points. These questions test the temporal lobes. *Total 7 points.*

Questions on Proverbs and Similarities

The person is asked to interpret two proverbs, a commonly used proverb and an unusual proverb. This tests the person's ability to conceptualize and think. The proverbs are: "A bird in the hand is worth two in the bush," and "a golden hammer breaks an iron door."

The person is asked how two seemingly different things are alike. A person with dementia will focus on the similarities, not the differences. The questions are: "How are a chicken and a duck alike?" and "How are an eye and ear alike?" These questions test the frontal lobes, a target of the dementia of PD. *Total 4 points.*

Questions on Following Commands, Sequencing, and Telling Right from Left

The person is asked to do the following:

- "If I clap once — you raise your right hand."
- "If I clap twice — you raise your left hand."
- "If I clap once — you cover your eyes."
- "If I clap twice — you cover your ears."
- Repeat after me, "No if's, ands, or buts about it."
- Name as many words, not proper names, as you can that begin with the letter "A."
- Name as many words as you can that begin with the letter "B."
- Name as many words as you can that begin with the letter "C."

(You must name at least five words with "A," "B," "C" to receive 1 point for "A," "B," "C.")

These questions test the frontal lobes and the language centers on the left side of the brain. (*Total 8 points.*)

Questions on Money and Arithmetic

The person is asked the following:

- How many nickels are there in a dollar? In three dollars?
- How many quarters are there in a dollar? In five dollars?
- If you have 28 quarters how many dollars do you have? How many nickels?

These questions test the frontal lobes, and the arithmetical skills of the right side of the brain. (*Total 4 points.*)

Questions on Visual Spatial Orientation

The person is asked to pick out the object that best fits a particular pattern. This tests the analytical skills of the frontal, parietal, and occipital lobes. (*Total 2 points.*) (See Figure 9.1.)

The PMMSE, like the MMSE, has 30 Points, but tests different parts of the brain. The PMMSE complements the Quality of Life Examination. The MMSE and the PMMSE are partly helpful in diagnosing dementia. But dementia may also be accompanied by daytime drowsiness (see Chapter 7) and psychosis (see below).

The following is a typical case history of a PD person with dementia.

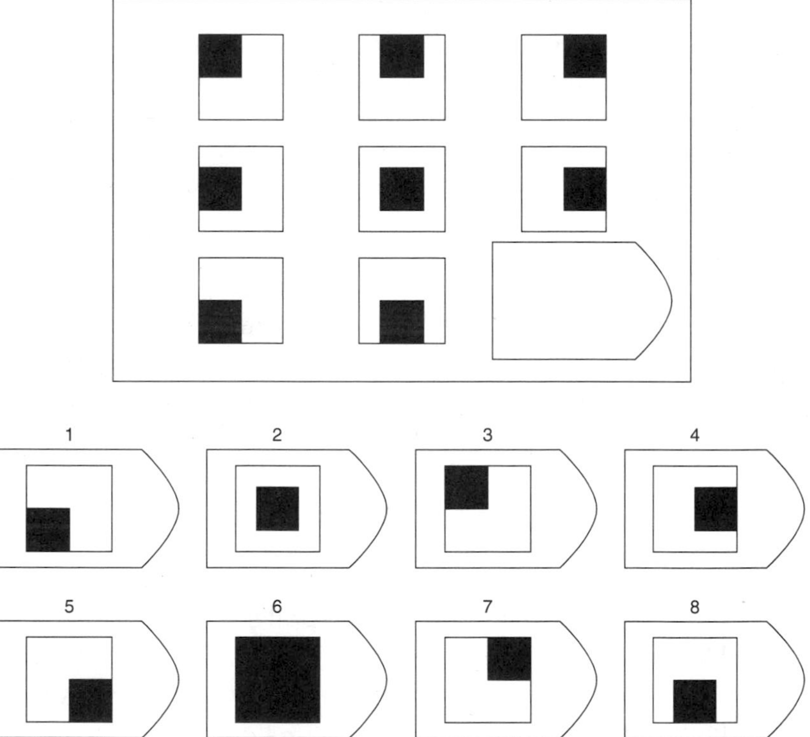

***Figure 9.1** Visual Spacial Orientation Exercise*
Which of Tabs 1–8 best fits the blank?

George, a 75-Year-Old Man with Parkinson and Dementia

George, my husband, was 70 years old when he was diagnosed with PD. George is a tennis player and was having difficulty with his backstroke. Recently he'd fallen and injured his right shoulder so we thought George's difficulty was related to the injury. Our doctor said it wasn't, he thought it was a nerve injury. I decided George had to see a neurologist. George is a visionary, he has the imagination to see things others can't, the drive to find the resources to develop them, and the organizational skills to make them go. George is enormously successful. And he's generous. He endowed a Chair at the University. So when I called the chairman of neurology, he saw us that day. The chairman examined George and thought he had a stroke. He ordered blood tests, an MRI of the brain, an MRA of George's blood vessels, and a consultation with a cardiologist. George, an engineer, was fascinated with the technology behind the tests. He forgot he was a patient, not an investor. Everything was normal, and the chairman said you can have a small stroke, and not be able to see anything on any of the tests. I was relieved because if it was a small stroke, the arm would get better.

When George's arm became worse, I became alarmed. My daughter-in-law, Kathy, is a nurse, a cancer nurse, and she explained that occasionally a brain tumor can start like a stroke. But whereas a stroke improves a tumor doesn't. I made an appointment with the chairman and he put George through all the tests again, and when they were normal we were puzzled. In retrospect, I should have appreciated that George didn't seem to care, he was passive — not a feature of George's personality.

Kathy's mother, Anna, has PD and Kathy insisted George see a PD specialist. It was awkward for the PD specialist, a junior member of the department seeing George, after George had been seen by the chairman. But Kathy and I were concerned for George, not the department chairman's ego. The specialist diagnosed PD — immediately. George refused treatment, his symptoms weren't troubling to him. And he could live without playing tennis.

I wanted George to retire, and he did. "When," I should've asked myself, "did George ever listen to me without arguing." Now George seemed depressed, he was apathetic, he lost interest in his hobbies, in thinking about things, in me. But George denied he was depressed, and he pointed out that if he was depressed, he wasn't depressed the way he was when his mother died. When his mother died, he was anxious, restless, and he cried. And he kept blaming himself for not doing more for his mother. The PD specialist called George's mood an apathetic depression and he tried several antidepression medications. None seemed to help.

Two years went by. And George began to stumble. And all of us, except George, thought it was time for treatment. The PD specialist recommended Sinemet, and then, Sinemet plus Comtan. George and I are religious, we read the Bible, we believe in God and in miracles. And Sinemet plus Comtan was a miracle. In a few weeks George was back to where he'd been before he injured his shoulder. He could play tennis, and he no longer seemed depressed. The next two years were a second honeymoon, literally and figuratively. The Sinemet, and later, Sinemet plus Comtan worked effectively and seamlessly. Then George fell and broke his right hip. Fixing the hip was a simple operation without complication. But as soon as George woke up from the anesthesia he was a "wild man": delusional, hallucinating, agitated. In retrospect it was the unmasking of his dementia.

The specialist reduced George's medication from four to three times a day. George was George again, except he couldn't walk as well. A year later George became apathetic. And now he slept most of the day. When the specialist increased George's medication back to four times a day, he perked up. Within a month, however, he was having nightmares. Next he accused me of having an affair with the specialist. I'm 70 years old, I never had sex with anyone but George. Then he accused me of poisoning him, and refused to take his pills. And then he began seeing people who were long dead: my mother, his mother, his father and all of them were fighting with him. "Is this," I asked the specialist, "dementia?"

"It could be," he replied. "But George is so irrational, psychotic, and wild from the medication I can't test his ability to think. Let's reduce his medication and place him on Clozaril. It's used to treat the psychosis of schizophrenia. And, unlike similar medications, it doesn't worsen the PD."

The psychosis cleared but George wasn't George. He couldn't think as imaginatively, as logically, and as constructively as before. And he slept all day. The specialist gave George the MMSE, and George, who had an

IQ of 175, scored 23, which is dementia. I don't know what George's IQ would've been, because at this stage he wasn't capable of taking an IQ test. The specialist placed George on Exelon. It's used in Alzheimer disease. "The dementia of PD," said the specialist, "is a cousin to the dementia of Alzheimer. And Exelon may help."

Exelon helped. George didn't sleep as much. And we could talk. It's difficult for me and our family dealing with dementia, more difficult than PD. But, and it's a blessing, it's not as difficult for George. He doesn't know he's demented. I love George, and I'm glad I have him and have the means to care for him. And I believe from this good will come. I answered the questions on the Quality of Life for George. After all it's as much my Quality of Life as it's George's.

George's Mobility Index is 25 (out of 40 points).

George's Emotional Index, and mine, is 23 (out of 44 points).

George's Autonomic Index is 7 (out of 16 points).

George's Total Score on the Quality of Life Scale is 55%.

I consider our Quality of Life as good, a gift from God.

I read the Bible daily to George. I quote from the Book of Wisdom.

WHO CAN KNOW GOD'S MIND? WHO CAN COMPREHEND GOD'S WILL?
FOR OUR REASONING IS SHALLOW, AND OUR MINDS ARE SHAKY
A PERISHABLE BODY CORRUPTS OUR SOUL, AND A TENT OF CLAY WEIGHS DOWN OUR MIND
IF IT'S HARD TO KNOW WHAT'S ON EARTH,
HOW THEN CAN WE KNOW WHAT'S IN HEAVEN?

The Anatomy of Dementia

The Dementia of Parkinson Disease

In PD there's a loss of nerve cells in the substantia nigra and locus ceruleus (two separate regions in the brainstem). This loss is associated with Lewy bodies, globs of protein, within the dying cells. In life, people with Lewy bodies in the brainstem have symptoms of PD. In the dementia of PD, in addition to Lewy bodies in the brainstem, there are Lewy bodies in the brain. People with Lewy bodies in the brainstem and brain may start with the symptoms of PD and then the symptoms of dementia, or they may start with the symptoms of PD and dementia, or they may start with the symptoms of dementia. In the last case they're diagnosed as having Dementia with Lewy Bodies or Diffuse Lewy Body Disease (abbreviated DLBD). This is assumed by most, but not all, doctors to be part of PD.

The Dementia of Alzheimer Disease

In Alzheimer disease, in contrast to PD, there's a loss of nerve cells in the brain: in the frontal, parietal, and temporal lobes. The cell loss is associated with ameba-like structures, called senile plaques, outside the cells. The plaques consist of a glob of amyloid (a protein) surrounded by distorted nerve fibers. Inside some dying cells there are other twisted and tangled nerve fibers. Many of these fibers contain globs of a protein called tau. Some dying nerve cells contain Lewy bodies that contain globs of at least three proteins: alpha synuclein, parkin, and ubiquitin.

The Dementia of Diffuse Lewy Body Disease

It was thought Diffuse Lewy Body Disease was uncommon. However, using newer methods it is estimated that among the four million people diagnosed with Alzheimer disease, 25%, or one million people, have Dementia with Lewy Bodies. If Dementia with Lewy Bodies is part of the spectrum of PD, then there are at least two million people with PD: half beginning as PD, and half beginning as dementia.

Drugs and Dementia

Until recently, dementia has been an unspoken secret of PD. The attitude was, "Why tell a person who's been diagnosed with PD he's at risk for dementia? At present, there's no treatment for dementia. And it's possible the person will die of the complications of PD before he develops dementia." But as the treatment of PD improved, as people lived longer, they developed dementia, a dementia they wouldn't have developed if the drugs for PD didn't enable them to live longer. Often, almost ungratefully, people ask, "Do the drugs for PD cause dementia?" No! In people who are "incubating" a dementia, some of the drugs may cause delusions and hallucinations. Although these side effects disappear when the drug is stopped they are a warning, a storm cloud. The storm may never come, but the cloud is bothersome. At present, there is no drug that will delay the dementia of PD. But if history's a guide, in the next few years such drugs will become available.

Sticky Proteins and Dementia

The dementia of PD, like PD itself, results from a deposit of proteins, proteins that have been changed, to become sticky and clump together. The process of getting sticky is only now being understood. Age is a factor. Proteins are made every day by the machinery of each brain cell. As each cell ages, the machinery inside ages, and the products the machines turn out aren't as pure as when the cell was young. Some of the proteins have defects, and in time the defects multiply, and the protein becomes sticky and clumps. This further clogs up the machinery of the cell. This is similar to, but different in detail, from Alzheimer disease. Understanding PD will lead to an understanding of Alzheimer, and vice versa. Two drugs, , Exelon and Aricept, are helpful in managing people with Alzheimer disease. Exelon and Aricept block the breakdown of acetyl choline, a naturally occurring chemical that regulates memory. Although not formally tested, Exelon and Aricept appear to be helpful in people with PD and dementia.

The "Psychosis" of Parkinson

Psychosis Is Not Dementia

Think of psychosis, abnormal or unusual behavior, as a blend of several primary colors including hallucinations, delusions, agitation, rage, and mood swings. The psychosis may consist of one, two, or more of the above primary colors. Psychosis occurs in 30% of PD people, some of whom develop dementia. Psychosis may precede the appearance of dementia, occur at the same time, or follow the appearance of dementia. In PD, psychosis usually results from either the occurrence of a condition such as an infection, a brain injury, or surgery. Or, more commonly, psychosis results from the effects of a PD drug. This is more so in older people who, knowingly or unknowingly, are suffering from an intellectual decline. In such people the PD drug results in overstimulation of the dopamine receptors causing psychosis. In PD, psychosis and dementia, more than an inability to walk, are responsible for nursing home placement. Of each 100 PD people who enter a nursing home, 80 do so because of psychosis and dementia, 20 because they can't walk.

Treating Psychosis

If psychosis appears, your doctor will search for a cause, and if possible, correct it. If the cause is a PD drug, or drugs, one or more will be stopped. Your doctor will start with the drugs that have the most potential for causing psychosis: the anticholinergics, amantadine, selegiline, and the dopamine agonists. Sinemet has the least potential for causing psychosis and usually can't be stopped or reduced without worsening PD. If the psychosis continues your doctor will add an antipsychosis drug, an atypical neuroleptic. The typical neuroleptics, Thorazine and Haldol, block dopamine receptors in all brain regions, preventing dopamine from stimulating the dopamine receptors — reducing psychosis. However, they can worsen PD and cause dyskinesias.

The atypical neuroleptics, Clozaril and Serequel, block dopamine receptors in selected brain regions, they don't worsen PD or cause dyskinesias. Clozaril is the more effective drug, but because in a small number of people it may drop the blood count, its use requires frequent blood tests. Serequel is not as effective, but does not require blood tests. Over 80% of PD people with psychosis respond to

Clozaril, with partial or complete disappearance of psychosis. The starting dose is 6.25 to 12.5 mg once or twice daily, increased by 12.5 mg every four to seven days until symptoms are reduced or disappear. Most people need a total dose of 12.5 mg to 37.5 mg per day. Clozaril and Serequel promote sleep at night. But both can cause daytime drowsiness, and Clozaril can cause a drop in blood pressure upon standing. Clozaril and Serequel, by reducing psychosis without worsening PD, have allowed many PD people to remain at home, avoiding placement in a nursing home.

In the past, a "drug holiday," withdrawal of all PD drugs, was used to treat a PD psychosis. However, the complications of a drug holiday — pneumonia, blood clots in the legs, and a condition called the malignant neuroleptic syndrome (high fever, muscle spasms, muscle breakdown, and kidney failure) — limited the usefulness of the holiday.

The following are the more common features of PD psychosis.

Hallucinations Are Not Dementia

(This was adapted from an article in the *NPF Parkinson Report* by Dr. Chris Goetz.)

In PD, hallucinations are usually caused by drugs, especially if the person has or is incubating a dementia. Sometimes hallucinations may occur in PD people not on drugs and may be a symptom of Diffuse Lewy Body Disease. In PD, in the absence of dementia, hallucinations occur in two ways.

1. A condition such as dehydration, infection, liver or kidney failure, a head injury, a surgical procedure, a drug for another disease (a disease other than PD), sleep deprivation, or alcohol withdrawal may be superimposed on PD, causing hallucinations. Such people are agitated, confused, and delusional in addition to having hallucinations.
2. PD drugs can cause hallucinations. The hallucinations consist of seeing things (visual hallucinations),

> feeling things (tactile hallucinations), hearing things (auditory hallucinations), or smelling things (olfactory hallucinations) that are not there. The hallucinations can occur in the absence of agitation or confusion or as part of a psychosis.

The hallucinations, confusion, agitation, and delusions in the first instance have no connection to PD, disappear when the conditions are corrected, and are of little further concern except for the need to alert new doctors to their occurrence and the circumstances of their occurrence. This can prevent or minimize their future occurrence. The hallucinations or psychosis in the second instance are of concern because they limit the use of these drugs for PD.

Most hallucinations consist of seeing things that do not exist, including recognizable or strange people (living or dead), animals, and objects. In 70% of people, the hallucinations are friendly or nonthreatening. In 30% of people the hallucinations are frightening. Most people realize they are seeing things that are not real. Yet they'll speak to them, invite them to sit down, or chase them away. Visual hallucinations are more common at night or in dim lighting. In some people they may be part of a vivid dream, continuing after they awake. Vivid dreams may, or may not, be a forerunner of hallucinations.

Hallucinations occur after PD people have been on drugs for years. If they appear after starting a new PD drug, this can indicate a sensitivity to the drug, or a disease such as Diffuse Lewy Body Disease rather than PD.

The Hallucination Questionnaire

This questionnaire was developed by me as a teaching aide for people with PD, their families, and doctors. The questionnaire has not been scientifically validated. It is not a substitute for a visit with your doctor.

THE HALLUCINATION QUESTIONNAIRE

If a hallucination, a false vision, occurred in the last week, answer the following:

1.	At night, did you see people, animals, or objects, no one else could see?	Yes	No
2.	Were they frightening?	Yes	No
3.	Did you talk to them?	Yes	No
4.	Did they talk back?	Yes	No
5.	During the day did you see people, animals, or objects, no one else could see?	Yes	No
6.	Were they frightening?	Yes	No
7.	Did you talk to them?	Yes	No
8.	Did they talk back?	Yes	No
9.	Did you think the people, animals, or objects were real?	Yes	No
10.	Did you feel insects, snakes, or anything else crawling on you?	Yes	No

Delusions

Delusions, believing false events are true or believing events that never happened happened, may occur in PD people. The delusions usually begin at night and may occur with hallucinations. How do you know a belief is a delusion — a false event? An event that never happened? One or two of the beliefs described below could be true. Perhaps people are stealing from you. Perhaps a 70-year-old spouse is, for the first time, having an affair. But three or more such beliefs are usually false — they are delusions. Delusions may arise from PD drugs, from depression, from anxiety, from difficulty sleeping, and from heavy drinking or withdrawal from alcohol.

The Delusion Questionnaire

This questionnaire was developed by me as a teaching aide. It hasn't been scientifically validated. It's not a substitute for a visit with your doctor.

THE DELUSION QUESTIONNAIRE

If a delusion occurred in the last week, answer the following:

1.	Did you believe people were planning to hurt you?	Yes	No
2.	Did you believe people were stealing from you?	Yes	No
3.	Did you believe your spouse was having an affair?	Yes	No
4.	Did you believe uninvited guests were living in your home?	Yes	No
5.	Did you believe your spouse wasn't who she or he said they were?	Yes	No
6.	Did you believe your home was not your home?	Yes	No
7.	Did you believe your family was planning to abandon you?	Yes	No
8.	Did you believe people were always saying bad things about you?	Yes	No
9.	Did you believe characters from a TV show were living in your home?	Yes	No
10.	Did they talk to you?	Yes	No

Rage

Rage is from the Latin *rabies* and means to go berserk, insane, or mad like a rabid dog. Rage is a blend of anger, agitation, and violence. *Anger* is from Latin and is related to anxiety and means to cause distress. *Agitation* is from Latin and means constant movement. *Violence* is from Latin and means to use force. Rage can be a combination of anger and agitation, or anger and violence, or agitation and violence, or anger, agitation, and violence. A rage attack is a burst of rage, a temporary burst of insanity or madness. Rage equivalents, words used in place of rage with different shades of meaning, include delirium, fit, frenzy, fury, mania, temper-tantrum, and uproar. Rage can be part of a psychosis. Rage can be part of dementia. Rage can occur in special circumstances or situations — situational rage — especially in people who are anxious, depressed, or are prone to having rage attacks. Situational rage includes air rage provoked, for example, by a plane sitting on a runway for hours and by you drinking heavily, or road rage provoked, for example, by sitting in a traffic jam, or being cut off in traffic.

The Rage Questionnaire

This questionnaire was developed by me as a teaching aide. It hasn't been scientifically validated. It's not a substitute for a visit with your doctor.

THE RAGE QUESTIONNAIRE

If rage occurred in the last week, answer the following questions. Indicate the time, place, and situation of the rage.

Verbal Rage

1.	Did you curse, scream, shout, or make threats?	Yes	No
2.	Before the rage were you angry?	Yes	No
3.	Before the rage were you jumpy?	Yes	No
4.	Before or during the rage were you driven or possessed?	Yes	No
5.	Before, during, or after the rage were you confused?	Yes	No

Rage at People, Animals, or Objects

6.	Did you spit at, grab, hit, injure, or kick anyone or anything?	Yes	No
7.	Before the rage were you angry?	Yes	No
8.	Before the rage were you jumpy?	Yes	No
9.	Before or during the rage were you driven or possessed?	Yes	No
10.	Before, during, or after the rage were you confused?	Yes	No

Self Rage

11.	Did you hit, injure, or kick yourself?	Yes	No
12.	Before the rage were you angry?	Yes	No
13.	Before the rage were you jumpy?	Yes	No
14.	Before or during the rage were you driven or possessed?	Yes	No
15.	Before, during, or after the rage were you confused?	Yes	No

Rage at Objects

16.	Did you spit at, break, hit, kick, or throw an object?	Yes	No
17.	Before the rage were you angry?	Yes	No
18.	Before the rage were you jumpy?	Yes	No
19.	Before or during the rage were you driven or possessed?	Yes	No
20.	Before, during, or after the rage were you confused?	Yes	No

Mood Swings

Mood swings, volatility, and emotional ups and downs in PD can be associated with fluctuations in response to PD drugs (see Chapter 10), anxiety, depression, difficulty sleeping, and dementia.

The Mood Swings Questionnaire

This questionnaire was developed by me as a teaching aide. It hasn't been scientifically validated. It's not a substitute for a visit with your doctor.

THE MOOD SWINGS QUESTIONNAIRE

If mood swings occurred in the last week, answer the following questions. Indicate the time, place, and situation of the mood swing.

1.	Were you calm one moment and agitated the next?	Yes	No
2.	Were you pleased one moment and angry the next?	Yes	No
3.	Were you happy one moment and miserable the next?	Yes	No
4.	Were you kind one moment and cruel the next?	Yes	No
5.	Were you self-assured one moment and doubting the next?	Yes	No
6.	Were you patient one moment and impatient the next?	Yes	No
7.	Were you gentle one moment and violent the next?	Yes	No
8.	Were you logical one moment and illogical the next?	Yes	No
9.	Were you laughing one moment and crying the next?	Yes	No
10.	Were you generous one moment and cheap the next?	Yes	No

Long-Term Care

Why Long-Term Care?

(This section was written with Ruth Hagestuen RN, Susan Imke RN, and Mary Willis.)

Long-term care is discussed here because dementia and psychosis are responsible for PD people considering it. Long-term care is defined as medical, nursing, rehabilitation, and support services provided outside the home for an indefinite time. This section is for the spouse and family of the PD person because, invariably, you will make the decision about long-term care. When should you begin to plan for long-term care? When your spouse is diagnosed with PD. It is depressing, but until a cure is found, it is necessary. The cost of long-term care insurance and your chance of obtaining it decreases as your need for it approaches. Sometime, in a calm moment, after your family has adjusted to PD, discuss long-term care — with your family, financial planner, insurance agent, and lawyer. If you never need it — great. If you need it — better ready than sorry.

Why Not Home Care?

Home care works well in moderately advanced PD. Home care can with ingenuity, imagination, or money work in advanced PD as in Lenny from Chapter 5, or in George from Chapter 9. But without George's resources, home care for the PD person with dementia is a full-time, physically and emotionally draining job: one that results in care-partner strain. If you do it without help and resources you, your spouse, and your family will burn out. Unless you are Superman or Wonder Woman, and unless your children are saints, you'll find yourself neglecting or quarreling with them. Lifting your spouse, taking your spouse to and from the bathroom, preparing meals, cleaning up after your spouse, giving your spouse medication, and worrying about your spouse's health is exhausting — and unhealthy.

If your spouse is up all night — so are you. But if he sleeps during the day — you won't. Sleep deprivation increases anxiety, depression, and rage in your spouse (and you). The person you are sacrificing everything for may be unappreciative or resentful of your sacrifice. As he absorbs himself in his disease, as he becomes unable to deal with it, he'll rage at you.

If your children are far away, as many are, they may not be able to help. And perhaps to ease their guilt, some long distance children will make up in advice for what they cannot give in care. And their advice, although well meaning, may be counter-productive and irritating. There are few people like Barbara: Jack Sr.'s daughter and caregiver, Jack Jr.'s sister and caregiver, and Dan's wife and caregiver. And you, unable to control your spouse's disease, or your life, may come to resent being controlled by your spouse, even though you love him. Such resentment leads to anger, guilt, depression, shame, and rage.

Children and Home Care

Susan Imke, a nurse practitioner speaks.

I arrange family conferences in which the goal is to make a decision about long-term care. Often, after everyone's agreed that home care is destroying both parents, it's the long distance son or daughter who voices the strongest opinion, "Put dad in a nursing home? Never!"

"Will you come and help?" I ask.

"I'd like to but I can't," replies the long distance son.

Susan adds, "I tell families to never make promises that may be impossible to keep. Rather than say, "Dad, we'll never put you in a nursing home," say, "We'll keep you at home as long as we can, and we won't make any decisions without asking you."

Mary Willis, NPF Coordinator, whose mother and father had PD, speaks.

I see problem after problem with a long distance son or daughter who appears "like a whirlwind" giving advice and dictating changes in a well worked-out and carefully established care plan. Such advice often leaves everyone, except the whirlwind, confused and upset.

But a long distance son or daughter, one not struggling with the grinding work of everyday care often has an overall perspective, an ability to "see the forest for the trees." But this perspective must be expressed diplomatically and without harsh criticism for those giving most of the on-going daily care.

Ruth Hagestuen RN, speaks on how long-distance children can help, short of moving back home.

Pick a time to call home each week and don't assume "no news is good news." Many older parents keep their own counsel even when times are tough, because they don't want to bother their grown-up children who are "busy with their own lives." Make the call and pay for it. It is amazing how many people, from a generation when a long-distance call costs more than a local call, shy away from making such calls. And while your mom and dad may love their daughter-in-law, or their son-in-law, and be glad to talk to them, it's you they want to talk with.

Ask tactfully but unequivocally whether your parents need financial help. Many parents won't ask for such help even when they need it. If a regular subsidy is unacceptable, offer something specific. If their insurance doesn't pay for drugs, offer to pay.

Send a surprise package once a month. This might be a bouquet of flowers, a restaurant gift certificate, or a basket of fruit. Even a card with an upbeat hand-written message means something during a hard day.

Make regular trips to check on your parents. And don't add to your parents' strain by expecting them to take care of you. Get your own ride from the airport. If crowded quarters are a strain, reserve a nearby hotel room. You aren't there to be entertained, but to provide a sympathetic ear and a helping hand.

Learn about PD and the drugs for PD. Go with your parents to see the doctor. What he says and what your parents say he says may not be the same. You may not be able to judge how much the doctor knows about PD, but you can judge how well he and his staff communicate with you and your parents.

Don't neglect your "well" parent. Ask your mom if she went for her mammography. Or if your dad went for his prostate exam.

Once or twice a year provide a 4- to 7-day respite for your caregiving parent. Plan to arrive a day or two before the caregiver's "leave of absence" so you can learn how to help your PD parent. If you can't fill-in personally, pay for a respite stay.

Remember them in your prayers, and tell them you do so.

Help for Home Care

If you're struggling to keep your spouse at home, many services can help. Some are covered by insurance, many are not. Don't ask yourself, "Is it covered?" Ask yourself, "Is it necessary?" If it will make you and your spouse's life easier — do it. If your spouse keeps you awake at night, hire a companion. If it's not covered — pay for it, the way you'd pay for staying in a hotel. Because if you can't sleep and have a nervous breakdown, where's the savings?

The following services are available in most communities. You can find them through the Yellow Pages, on the Internet at **www. parkinson.org,** your NPF support group, or a social worker:

1. Companions who will read to your spouse, sit with your spouse, or stay with your spouse while you sleep. These services are usually not covered by insurance.
2. Housekeeping services that will clean your house (not your spouse), shop for you, prepare or deliver meals for you ("meals on wheels"), and run errands. Most of these services are not covered by insurance, but some are subsidized by charitable or community groups.
3. Adult day care provides personal care, exercise, physical therapy, social activities, discussion groups, arts and crafts, hobbies, games, and meals. Adult day care complements living at home. Adult day care may be sponsored by a hospital, a senior center, a local PD support group, or other agency. The seniors are usually disabled. Respite care allows you a few hours a day to yourself. There are differences in meaning from state to state between adult day care and respite care and who pays for it. Ask about the differences.

   Senior centers offer organized programs, activities, outings, and companionship, usually at no cost for seniors who are not disabled.
4. Home health care, through a charity or a local hospital, provides in-home services by nurses, physical therapists, dietitians, and other medical professionals. Depending upon the type of problem, and the nature of the service, insurance may cover home health care, or it may cover it partly, or for a defined period of time. There are many well-managed and ethical home health care services, but as a rule it is

best to deal with a nonprofit agency. There's less motivation to provide services that are not needed, and they are more likely to be up front about costs.

5. Rehabilitation provides physical therapy, occupational therapy, and speech therapy. These may be provided at home or in a facility. Depending upon the disease, and the nature of the rehabilitation needed, insurance may pay for it. Your doctor must approve such services.
6. Retirement communities offer living quarters, building security, and social activities. Depending on the community, they may provide medical personnel to assist you. Retirement communities were not specifically designed for the disabled. If you were living in a retirement community before your spouse was diagnosed with PD, you won't be asked to leave. But if your spouse has been diagnosed and is disabled, you may have difficulty moving into some communities.
7. Assisted living offers everything retirement communities offer plus medical attention, as well as assistance with eating, bathing, and other activities of daily living. Many retirement communities offer assisted living. It is not the home you lived in all your married life, but you are together, there's help all around. Assisted living isn't cheap, and it is not covered by insurance. But it is usually worth the cost.

Long-Term Care

No Guilt, No Regret

When you got married, when he developed PD, you promised each other "never a nursing home." Now your family has concluded that a nursing home is best. Everyone is guilt-stricken, bitter about the broken promise, and terrified by horror stories of nursing homes. Know this, in the past people with PD did not live as long as they do today. The drugs that control their symptoms and let them live do not halt the progression of PD. And today, people with PD (or Alzheimer disease) develop problems not seen in the past — because they're living longer. Lenny in Chapter 2, because of his physical disability, and George in Chapter 9, because of his mental disability, need at least one person every eight hours to provide care. And to lift Lenny, or bathe George, two people are needed.

How many of you have Lenny's or George's resources? It is estimated that 95% of you don't have these resources. The decision to place your spouse in a home is one not to "make your life more comfortable" but to make "his life more comfortable." Nursing homes offer 24-hour, round-the-clock services. Nursing homes offer two or more people to bathe your spouse. And nursing homes don't fall apart when someone who was supposed to show up at midnight does not.

Studying the Nursing Home

Determine the level of care your spouse needs. Your doctor, your spouse's nurse, physical therapist, occupational therapist, or social worker can determine this. And they can usually recommend several homes in your community, ones you can visit easily.

Study the services of the different homes in your community. How are they rated? Most states that license nursing homes also rate them. If the home isn't rated, check the home's inspection results when you visit. The rating should be posted near the home's license.

Examine the quality and skill of the staff. You may not be able to evaluate their professional skill, but you can evaluate their interpersonal skills. And if there's a question about their professional skill bring a family member who can help you evaluate. The nursing home should have registered nurses (RNs), licensed practical nurses (LPNs), and nurses' aids, who work around-the-clock (most often in eight-hour shifts). Ask about the ratio of RNs, the most highly trained (and expensive), to LPNs and nurses' aids. This usually sets the level of care. Ask about services your spouse may need such as physical, occupational, speech, or respiratory therapy. Are they part of the program or do you pay extra?

Ask about staff turnover. If the turnover is high it may mean the staff is underpaid, overworked, and — unhappy. If the turnover is high or if the home uses too many temporary workers hired from outside to work a single shift, it means the staff won't get to know your spouse and give him the personalized care he needs.

Ask if there's a doctor on staff who's available for emergencies. Ask if he responds promptly. Ask the director of nursing for the name of the doctor. Then ask your family doctor about the home's doctor. If necessary visit the home's doctor. You may not be able to judge his professional skill, but you can judge his manner and his interpersonal skills. Don't expect him to be an expert on PD, he must know something about many diseases, he can't concentrate on one. But ask if he'll work with your family doctor and PD doctor. It is a red flag if he says, "No." And ask what hospital your spouse will go to in an emergency. If there's no formal affiliation with a hospital, or the hospital is not one you would choose, this is another red flag.

Ask if there's a social worker on staff. Social workers are licensed professionals who help residents and their families adjust to the move. They provide psychological and sociological counseling. They are usually caring, kind, and attentive — why else go into social work? Ask the social worker about the home's policies. Ask if you're notified immediately of an emergency. Can you see the care plan? Ask if restraints are used without telling you or the doctor. Ask if the home can or will accept Medicare, Medicaid, or your insurance as full or partial payment. If not, ask yourself if you can afford the home. Ask about "additional" or "hidden" costs, such as nutritional supplements, prescription and nonprescription drugs, hair cuts, laundry, doctors' visits, and cable TV.

Ask the social worker if the home requires a deposit to reserve a room. If so, find out if the deposit is refundable, and under what circumstances. Contracts vary from one home to another, and from state to state. There are two things that nursing homes cannot do because they are illegal. They cannot make you pay privately if your spouse is eligible for Medicaid. They cannot make you give a donation as a condition of admission.

If you can, if there's time, visit several nursing homes before making your choice. If you or your children went to college, you visited several schools, studied their programs, spoke to their professors and students, examined their facilities, and examined your finances. Could you afford it? An education was something you needed — and you paid for it. Medicare or Medicaid didn't pay for college. Choose a nursing home with the same care you used to choose a college: it is equally as important.

In this, a dark hour, do not forget the Bible, or God. Listen to Jeremiah.

> DISASTER IS NOT ME! WHAT A WOUND! MY INJURY IS INCURABLE.
> IF THIS IS THE WORST, I CAN BEAR IT!
> BUT NOW MY TENT IS DESTROYED, ALL MY CORDS ARE SNAPPED,
> MY SONS HAVE LEFT ME AND ARE NO MORE,
> NO ONE IS LEFT TO PUT MY TENT UP AGAIN.
> I KNOW GOD, NO ONE'S LIFE IS IN HIS CONTROL,
> BUT HELP ME, OH GOD!
> AND GOD ANSWERS,
> "LET THE SAGE NOT BOAST OF WISDOM, NOR THE VALIANT OF BRAVERY,
> NOR THE WEALTHY OF RICHES!
> BUT LET ANYONE WHO WANTS TO BOAST, BOAST OF THIS,
> OF UNDERSTANDING AND KNOWING GOD,
> FOR I AM GOD, WHO ACTS WITH FAITHFUL LOVE."

CHAPTER
10

Treating Parkinson — What Science Can Do

Pete, a 60-Year-Old Man with "On and Off"

I was diagnosed with PD eight years ago. Looking back, however, I realize I had it two years before. I wear a self-winding wristwatch and one day it stopped. The dealer said it was fine. When it stopped a second time I sent it to the factory. The factory said it was fine. When it stopped a third time I bought a battery-powered watch. Months later my wife noticed I wasn't swinging my left arm. Her father had PD and died 10 years ago at 75. He was diagnosed at 55 and lived 20 years with PD. A neurologist confirmed my wife's diagnosis: I had PD.

I knew things had changed in the 10 years since my father-in-law died. There were new ideas, new drugs. I contacted the National Parkinson Foundation and read their material. Then my wife and I discussed our options with our neurologist. I decided I could live with my symptoms: slowness and tremor of my left hand. I saw my neurologist regularly every four months. My wife and I can't see what our neurologist sees. And our neurologist knows firsthand the latest developments.

Two years later my tremor got worse and I dragged my left foot. My wife, our neurologist, and I, agreed I needed treatment. Sinemet, the drug my father-in-law used, was still the best drug. But to work it must be changed to dopamine in the brain. And as the number of specialized cells, the "factories" that change Sinemet into dopamine decrease, the remaining "factories" need a constant and uninterrupted supply of Sinemet. Temporary interruptions, inevitable as PD progresses, result in fluctuations: the "on-off" effect. Accompanying on-off are dyskinesias: twisting or jerking movements. We knew about on-off and dyskinesias from my father-in-law.

"To postpone on-off and dyskinesias," our neurologist said, "we're studying several different drugs that block an enzyme COMT that breaks down Sinemet, increasing Sinemet's duration of action. By starting drug therapy early, before on-off and dyskinesias begin, we may be able to postpone them in people with PD. That's why we're doing theses studies."

I started on Sinemet CR (controlled release, long-acting Sinemet) plus Comtan: one tablet of Sinemet 50/200 with one 200 mg tablet of Comtan twice a day. Comtan plus Sinemet CR worked well. My tremor stopped and my wristwatch restarted. Through the NPF we found a support group and attended regularly. Most of the people are like us, still working, putting their children through college, paying-down their mortgages. And worried about the future. But we're blessed with drugs we didn't have when my father-in-law was alive. Lenny and his wife, our support group leaders, are an inspiration. Lenny has a PD-like disease, Shy Drager, he's disabled but not depressed, angry, or bitter. And he wishes the drugs worked on him, no matter what they cost, as they worked on us.

It's 10 years after my wristwatch stopped running. It's eight years since I was diagnosed, six years since I started Comtan and Sinemet. And I'm having on-off. I'm doing better than my father-in-law: he began having on-off three years after he was diagnosed. When my medicine's working I'm "on," I'm normal. And I can do all of my necessary daily activities: shaving, bathing, dressing, and eating. When I'm "off," one or two 30-minute periods at day's end or during the night, I have trouble turning in bed, I get cramps in my calves, I have trouble getting out of a chair, and I have occasional "freezing spells" — periods of being unable to move for a few seconds.

Sometimes I'm depressed and anxious in my "off periods." Partly it's a feeling of helplessness, a loss of control. Partly it's rigidity, stiffness, of my chest muscles. These muscles act as a "bellows" and if they're rigid, I can't breath deeply. So I take shorter, shallower, more frequent breaths: I hyperventilate. And this makes me more anxious. And sometimes I panic, I think I'll never move again. From my therapist I learned how to beat hyperventilation and now I don't panic.

My father-in-law lived 20 years with PD on Sinemet alone. But I've done better with a longer acting drug: Sinemet CR plus Comtan. After all, despite having on-off periods my wristwatch is still running. I took the Quality of Life exam and although my mobility is compromised, I'm not.

My Mobility Index is 21 (out of 40 points).
My mobility is "off" when my medicine is not working.
My Emotional Index is 12 (out of 44 points).
My Autonomic Index is 9 (out of 16 points).
My Total Score on the Quality of Life Scale is 42%.
I consider my Quality of Life to be good.

What You Should Know About Drugs

Finding the right drug in the right dose can be difficult. Some people respond better to one drug than to another. And some people develop side effects on one drug and not another. Be active! Don't just take your pills. When you get a prescription, do the following:

1. Get the brand name and the generic name of the drug and the dose (in milligrams). Write it down. Telling a doctor "I take, two large blue pills" isn't helpful. There are hundreds of large, blue pills. If

you can't take the time to know what you're taking, why should the doctor?

2. Why am I taking this drug? Is it to replace another drug?
3. How will I know if the drug is working?
4. What are the side effects? Are they serious?
5. Can I drive or drink alcohol if I take the drug?
6. Are there any drugs I should not take if I take this drug?

Drugs are misused in many ways. The drug may not be taken as prescribed; you may skip a dose and "make it up" by taking an extra dose; you may "experiment" with a friend's drug; or your drugs may be outdated. (Note: Check the expiration date of every drug you take.)

The Time It Takes for the Drug to "Peak" In Your Blood

The time the drug takes to reach its peak concentration determines how fast the drug acts. The shorter the time to peak the faster acting the drug. A drug that peaks at half-an-hour means the drug acts four times as fast as a drug that peaks at 2 hours. As a rule, the faster to the peak, and the higher the peak, the more likely you'll notice the effect of the drug. Sinemet peaks in 30 minutes, which is why you can tell it is working.

The Time It Takes for the Drug to Be Eliminated from Your Body (Its Half-Life)

The half-life of a drug is the time it takes for a drug's peak concentration to be cut in half. As a rule it takes five half-lives for a drug to be eliminated and no longer have an effect. If the drug's half-life is four hours, then four hours after the drug has peaked half the drug has been eliminated. If the drug's peak concentration is 80 units, then four hours or one half-life later the drug's concentration is 40 units. Four hours or two half-lives later the drug's concentration is 20 units. Four hours or three half-lives later the drug's concentration is 10 units. Four hours or four half-lives later the drug's concentration is 5 units, and four hours or five half-lives later the drug's concentration is 2.5 units and no longer effective. How do we check progression of half-life? The drug's half-life is determined by how fast the drug is absorbed; how fast and completely it is metabolized in the liver; how fast it is excreted in the urine, through the lungs, or through skin (in the sweat); and how fast it is absorbed, stored, and released from depots in the muscle and fat. In addition, some drugs are metabolized and their breakdown products are as active as the original drug. For example, Elavil (an antidepression drug) is metabolized to Pamelor, also an antidepression drug.

Solubility

Drugs that are soluble in *lipids,* or fats, cross from the blood into the brain (through the "blood brain barrier"). Drugs that are insoluble in fats do not cross from the blood into the brain. This isn't surprising, as the brain is mainly made up of fat: highly specialized fat, but basically fat. Drugs that enter the brain may act differently from drugs that do not enter the brain. Think of the drugs as a stain. A drug whose base is water will stain tissue differently from a drug whose base is oil or fat. Which drugs are harder to predict? Turn the question around: "Which stains are harder to remove: water or oil?"

What Happens When You Don't Understand a Drug

An example of how a new and well-studied drug, Comtan, came to be misunderstood is illustrated. Comtan blocks an enzyme, COMT, that delays the breakdown of Sinemet, allowing more Sinemet to enter the brain. Comtan does not act alone; it must be combined with Sinemet. The benefits of Comtan are the benefits of Sinemet acting longer. The side effects of Comtan are similar to the side effects of Sinemet and can include dyskinesia, nausea, diarrhea, abdominal pain, and urine discoloration. The dyskinesia may improve after reduction of the Sinemet dose. Nonetheless, a year after Comtan became available, 20% of people taking Comtan didn't understand why they were taking it. Either it wasn't explained properly, or the explanation was misunderstood. The "Ask the Doctor" section on the NPF Web site (www.parkinson.org) received the following questions, multiple times.

Scenario A

PD person: "I started Comtan and it doesn't work."

Ask the Doctor replies: "How much Sinemet are you taking?"

PD person: "I stopped taking Sinemet."

Ask the Doctor replies: "Comtan acts in combination with Sinemet. Taken without Sinemet it has no effect."

Scenario B

PD person: "When should I take Comtan?"

Ask the Doctor replies: "For the best effect, if you are experiencing "on-off," you should take 200 mg of Comtan with each dose of Sinemet.

Scenario C

PD person: "If I take Comtan, can I substitute a dopamine agonist for Sinemet?"

Ask the Doctor replies: "Comtan does not prolong the action of an agonist, it prolongs the action of Sinemet. You can't substitute an agonist for Sinemet. But you can add an agonist to Comtan plus Sinemet."

Scenario D

PD person: "Does Comtan cause hallucinations?"

Ask the Doctor replies: "Comtan does not enter the brain, so Comtan, by itself, does not cause hallucinations. However, in some people, older people, when Comtan is added to Sinemet the combination may cause hallucinations. Don't stop Comtan, reduce Sinemet."

Scenario E

PD person: "Does Comtan cause dyskinesias?"

Ask the Doctor replies: "Comtan does not enter the brain, so Comtan, by itself, does not cause dyskinesias. However, in some people, when Comtan is added to Sinemet the combination may cause dyskinesias. Don't stop Comtan, reduce Sinemet."

Scenario F

PD person: "I've been taking Comtan and my urine is orange. Should I worry?"

Ask the Doctor replies: "In some people Comtan colors the urine orange. This is not a reason to worry."

Scenario G

PD person: "Will I need less Sinemet if I take Comtan?"

Ask the Doctor replies: "Comtan prolongs Sinemet's effect. If you have on-off without dyskinesias you won't need to reduce Sinemet. If you have on-off with dyskinesias you may need to reduce Sinemet."

Drugs That Increase Dopamine in the Brain

Levodopa

The main problem in PD is a loss of dopamine in the brain. Parkinson starts with a loss of dopamine producing cells (dopamine factories) in the substantia nigra. These cells supply dopamine to another region of the brain, the striatum, where dopamine is stored. These dopamine "stores" are shown on the PET Scan in Chapter 1. When 240,000 factories — 60% of the 400,000 cells in the substantia nigra — are lost, the symptoms of PD appear. At this time, when PD is diagnosed, the dopamine stores in the striatum are reduced by 80%.

Levodopa is supplied in the diet either as levodopa (in foods such as fava beans) or in tyrosine (an amino acid found in most dietary proteins). In the absence of PD, enough levodopa from the diet is able to enter the factories of the substantia nigra, be changed into dopamine, and be transported to the striatum where it is stored till needed. In PD, as the number of factories in the substantia nigra are reduced, the remaining factories cannot change, in an efficient way, the small amount of dietary levodopa to dopamine. These cells need an extra supply, "a boost." Levodopa in Sinemet is that boost. In Sinemet, levodopa is combined with carbidopa. The ratio is usually 4 mg of levodopa to 1 mg of carbidopa. The traditional Sinemet tablet is 25/100; the 25 is 25 mg of carbidopa, and the 100 is 100 mg of levodopa. Sometimes the ratio is 10 mg of levodopa to 1 mg of carbidopa, this is the Sinemet 10/100 or 25/250 tablet. The 10 or 25 is 10 or 25 mg of carbidopa, and the 100 or 250 is 100 mg or 250 mg of levodopa.

In Sinemet CR (controlled release) levodopa is combined with carbidopa and is fixed in a matrix that releases carbidopa and levodopa slowly, prolonging levodopa's effect. Comtan also prolongs levodopa's effect but in a different way, by blocking an enzyme, COMT, which breaks down levodopa. There are two forms of Sinemet CR, 50/200 and 25/100; the 25 or 50 is 25 or 50 mg of carbidopa, and the 100 or 200 is 100 or 200 mg of levodopa. Because of the way carbidopa and levodopa are combined in the Sinemet CR matrix, they are released differently from carbidopa and levodopa in Sinemet; the strengths of the drugs cannot be directly compared. Just as a "double" in baseball is not the equivalent of two "singles," so a Sinemet CR 50/200 is not the equivalent of two Sinemet 25/100 tablets.

Levodopa without carbidopa is rapidly changed into dopamine in the body by an enzyme: dopa decarboxylase. This enzyme is present in the stomach, the liver, the kidneys, the blood vessels, and the brain. If levodopa is given without carbidopa, 99% of it is changed into dopamine in the stomach, the liver, the kidneys, and the blood vessels, and only 1% of it is available to the cells (factories) in the substantia nigra and the storage facilities in the striatum. And the dopamine that is produced by the stomach, the liver, and the kidneys causes nausea. Before carbidopa was combined with levodopa, the main side effect of levodopa was nausea. As many as half of the people with PD stopped taking levodopa because of nausea. Carbidopa combined with levodopa in a single tablet blocks Dopa Decarboxylase in the stomach, the liver, the kidneys, and the blood vessels. This allows almost 10% of a dose of levodopa to enter the brain. However, carbidopa itself cannot enter the brain. Look at carbidopa as Moses: he brought the Children of Israel to the Promised Land, the brain, but he himself could not enter it. In the brain, the added levodopa is changed to dopamine in the factories of the substantia nigra, and transported and stored in the striatum. Since little dopamine is produced in the stomach, the liver, and the kidney, nausea and vomiting is rarely a problem. Indeed the name, Sinemet, is from Latin "Sine" meaning *without,* and "emit" meaning *vomiting*. So Sinemet means *without vomiting* (or nausea).

Sinemet (Generic Carbidopa/Levodopa)

Dose

Sinemet: carbidopa to levodopa available in the following ratios: 10/100, 25/100, 25/250.

Starting dose, early PD, 25/100, two to three times a day.

In advanced PD, from four to eight times a day, to every two hours round-the-clock.

Sinemet CR: controlled release available in 25/100 and 50/200.

Starting dose, early PD, 50/200, two to three times a day.

In advanced PD, use as needed.

Side Effects

Nausea, loss of appetite, drop in blood pressure on standing — these are related to the effects of dopamine produced in the stomach, the liver, the kidneys, and the blood vessels. "Wearing-off" or "on-off" are related to continued loss of factories in the substantia nigra, with inability of the remaining factories to supply a constant amount of dopamine to the brain. In advanced PD, some levodopa may reach the striatum, not from the substantia nigra but through the blood vessels of the striatum. Such levodopa, which is changed to dopamine in the blood vessels, is probably more susceptible to breakdown and shorter lived. Think of the striatum as leaves on a tree. You can irrigate it with water that comes up from the roots and branches to reach the leaves (this is the route of levodopa from the substantia nigra). Or, you can irrigate the leaves by spraying them with water (this is the route of levodopa from blood vessels). Because the blood vessel levodopa is shorter lived, it is more necessary to prolong it with Comtan.

Dyskinesias are related to sensitization of the PD brain to the effects of levodopa, which is delivered not continuously, but intermittently. The brain "sees" and "feels" dopamine not as a continuous stream, but as a series of highs and lows. These lows may be responsible, in part, for dyskinesias. Hallucinations are related to the effects of levodopa on a brain whose thinking is altered by PD.

Interactions

Vitamin B6 (pyridoxine) 50 mg or more a day may decrease the effect of levodopa. Protein-rich meals, rich in amino acids such as valine, leucine, and isoleucine, may compete with levodopa for absorption from the stomach, or for transportation from the blood into the brain. About 20% of people with PD are sensitive to the effects of a protein-rich meal and "turn off" shortly after eating it. You can test if you are "protein sensitive" by taking Sinemet with a protein-rich meal. If you are "protein sensitive" you'll turn off shortly after you finish eating. If you're protein sensitive take Sinemet on an empty stomach an hour before you eat.

Sinemet and the Diagnosis of Parkinson

Sinemet is so effective that many doctors, uncertain of the diagnosis of PD, prescribe Sinemet. If after three months on Sinemet at a dose of at least 25/100 four times a day there is no effect, it is unlikely you have PD, rather you may have a PD-like disease.

Is Sinemet Bad?

In time, after five years, the effect of Sinemet seems to decrease. Sinemet is just as potent, but the brain is changed by PD. There are fewer factories in the substantia nigra, and they are less efficient at changing levodopa to dopamine. Any interruption in supply—from a protein-rich meal to missing a dose of Sinemet—results in turning "off." Comtan, when added to Sinemet in patients having on-off, increases Sinemet's availability and helps reduce "off" time. In addition, five years after diagnosis, the brain has been sensitized by PD and by levodopa. Some of it may relate to changes in the dopamine receptors in the striatum, some of it may relate to the peaks and valleys or the highs and lows — especially the lows associated with Sinemet. None of it relates to a toxic effect of Sinemet, or to a destruction of cells by Sinemet.

In some PD people, a more continuous flow of dopamine to the brain is helpful. This might be accomplished by adding Comtan to Sinemet, by adding a dopamine agonist, or by changing the brain through deep brain stimulation (DBS).

On-Off: It's Like a Light Switch

In a person with PD, starting Sinemet usually results in improvement. Symptoms may disappear and you may be unaware you have PD. This "Sinemet honeymoon" can last up to five years, perhaps longer with Sinemet plus Comtan. During this time, like Pete, you may not have on-off. However, eventually you may feel a decrease in your mobility or an increase in your tremor between doses of Sinemet. This is the "wearing-off" effect, a part of on-off.

Wearing off starts gradually. For example, you may wake up in the morning and find some of your PD symptoms are back. Or you may find some of your symptoms are back before your next dose of Sinemet. Or you may have a rapid and abrupt return of your PD symptoms. This last situation is the on-off effect. It's called on-off because it's like a light switch being turned on or off. Parkinson specialists use wearing off and on-off to refer to two different things. Most people with PD use them interchangeably. I use on-off to include wearing off and on-off. Remember, "on" is when Sinemet is working, and "off" is when it is not.

If you have on-off, complete the following questionnaire. It's a good way to work with your doctor to come up with the best treatment.

On-off Questionnaire

1. Recently, have you felt a difference in your response to your first dose of the day and later doses of the day of Sinemet?
2. Recently, have you increased the frequency of your doses of Sinemet?
3. Recently, have you felt your dose of Sinemet does not last as long?
4. Recently, have you felt you need Sinemet as soon as you wake up?
5. Recently, have you felt that if you take Sinemet during or after a big meal it doesn't work?
6. Recently, have you felt that missing a dose of Sinemet stops you from doing what you are doing?
7. Recently, have you felt that after taking Sinemet and exercising Sinemet doesn't work?
8. Recently, have you felt you must wake up in the middle of the night and take Sinemet?
9. Recently, do you become anxious or panic before your next dose of Sinemet?

   If you answered "Yes" to two or more of the above, you may be experiencing on-off.

Comtan

Dose

Comtan (Entacapone) is available only in 200 mg tablets. The recommended dose is one 200 mg tablet with each dose of Sinemet, up to eight Comtan tablets daily. In the beginning, you may start with 200 mg of Comtan with every other dose of Sinemet and gradually build up to a full dose of 200 mg of Comtan with each dose of Sinemet. Comtan does not work alone, only when combined with Sinemet (or generic carbidopa/levodopa). It works with Sinemet or Sinemet CR.

How Does Comtan Work?

Comtan works by blocking an enzyme, COMT. Taking 100 mg of Comtan does not block COMT. COMT is found throughout your body with the highest amounts in your liver and kidney. COMT also occurs in your heart, lung, and skeletal muscles. Comtan is a reversible blocker of COMT; its effects are over within four hours. Comtan does not enter the brain. The more frequently Sinemet plus Comtan is given, the more prolonged the effects of Sinemet. There is less on-off but more dyskinesias.

Comtan, alone, or with Sinemet, does not prolong the action of a dopamine agonist. However, Comtan plus Sinemet and a dopamine agonist can be used together. Especially if you have dyskinesias.

Side Effects

Comtan is generally well tolerated and does not require any specific safety monitoring. The most commonly reported side effects are dyskinesias, nausea, diarrhea, abdominal pain, and discoloration of urine.

Interactions

Comtan shouldn't be taken with an antidepression drug that blocks an enzyme MAO "A." Comtan may be taken with selegiline at doses up to 10 mg a day. (See Chapter 8).

When to Start Comtan

The decision on when to start Comtan must be discussed with your doctor. There is agreement that Comtan should start when on-off starts. There is evidence that Comtan prevents the "lows" of Sinemet and, therefore, perhaps it should be started when you start Sinemet.

By preventing the lows (low blood and, presumably low brain levels of Levodopa) of Sinemet, Comtan plus Sinemet may not only reduce on-off but delay the appearance of on-off.

Selegiline

Dose

Selegiline (Eldepryl) is given as a 5 mg tablet or capsule once or twice a day.

How Does Selegiline Work?

Selegiline works by blocking an enzyme, MAO "B." It takes 5 to 10 mg of selegiline to block MAO "B" for up to one month. There are two forms of MAO: MAO "A" and MAO "B," they are found in different regions of the brain and they break down different chemicals. MAO "A" breaks down serotonin, a chemical involved in depression. Drugs that block MAO "A" prolong the actions of serotonin and improve depression (see Chapter 8). Certain foods, aged cheese, and red wine, for example, contain a chemical tyramine. This is inactivated by MAO "A." If MAO "A" is blocked, tyramine is increased. This can result in an increase in blood pressure, and has led to heart attacks and strokes. People taking MAO "A" inhibitors (or blockers) are cautioned not to eat certain foods. Selegiline at a dose of 5 mg to 10 mg blocks MAO "B," not MAO "A." This prevents the break down of dopamine and prolongs its action. People on selegiline at a dose of 5 mg to 10 mg do not have to worry about eating certain foods.

Selegiline is an irreversible blocker of MAO "B," its effects persist for up to one month after it is stopped. This has nothing to do with selegiline's half-life; it has everything to do with its ability to block an enzyme. It takes about one month for the body to replace the MAO "B" that has been blocked. Selegiline used alone prolongs the action of the dopamine that your brain produces. Selegiline can be used by itself as a treatment for PD. It has a mild effect on PD. Selegiline can be combined with Sinemet or Sinemet CR. It prolongs the actions of Sinemet. Currently another MAO "B" blocker, rasagiline, is being studied in PD. Rasagiline is a reversible blocker of MAO "B," is a more specific blocker of MAO "B," and lacks an amphetamine effect. Selegiline has a mild amphetamine effect.

Side Effects

The side effects are similar to those of Sinemet. Selegiline is changed in part to amphetamine. There's a "D" and an "L" form of amphetamine. The "D" form is more active and is known on the street as "uppers." The "L" is the breakdown product of selegiline. Although it is less active, it can keep you awake, and selegiline should not be taken after 12 P.M. Occasionally people taking selegiline are screened for amphetamines and their urine is positive. Explain to the person who orders the test that you are on selegiline, not "uppers."

Drug Interactions

If you are on selegiline, a narcotic analgesic, such as demerol, shouldn't be taken. If you're going for surgery and will be receiving narcotics, you should stop selegiline at least two weeks before surgery.

There are interactions between MAO "A," tricyclic antidepression drugs and SSRIs. Although such interactions don't occur with MAO "B" blockers, caution is advised if you're on selegiline and need an antidepression drug.

Does Selegiline Stop Parkinson Disease?

It was thought selegiline, by blocking MAO "B," stopped the production of a chemical responsible for the progression of PD. Selegiline does block the production of the chemical, but the chemical isn't responsible for the progression of PD. Selegiline does not stop or delay the progression of PD.

The Dopamine Agonists

What Are Antagonists? What Are Agonists?

Dopamine antagonists are drugs used in schizophrenia and psychosis (Chapter 9). Dopamine antagonists bind to dopamine receptors. They stop dopamine from binding to and stimulating the receptor. And in so doing they prevent dopamine from acting. Agonists are the opposite of antagonists. Agonists also bind to dopamine receptors, stopping dopamine from binding to the receptor. But like dopamine, and unlike an antagonist, they stimulate the receptor. And in so doing they mimic the actions of dopamine.

What Are the Advantages of Agonists?

Because agonists do not have to be changed to dopamine by the decreasing number of dopamine factories in the substantia nigra, they are able to act continuously with fewer interruptions than Sinemet. In addition, the agonists currently available have a longer half-life than Sinemet. Thus, independently of the number of dopamine factories, they result in prolonged stimulation of the dopamine receptors. This results in a decrease in on-off, and a decrease in dyskinesias.

What are the Disadvantages of the Agonists?

Although the agonists are longer acting, they are not as potent as Sinemet. They don't reduce the symptoms of PD as completely as Sinemet. There are five dopamine receptors in the brain: D-1, D-2, D-3, D-4, and D-5. The D-1 and D-2 receptors are relevant for PD. The D-3 receptor may be relevant for anxiety or depression. The roles of D-4 and D-5 are being studied. Sinemet stimulates both D-1 and D-2. The agonists stimulate mainly D-2. Stimulation of D-1 may be responsible for Sinemet's added potency. It may also be responsible, in part, for dyskinesia. The agonists must be started slowly to circumvent side effects (nausea, a drop in blood pressure), and built up over several days or weeks to full effect. Older people, or people with a decline in intellect, are more likely to have hallucinations on an agonist than on Sinemet.

In some people agonists (and Sinemet) can cause daytime drowsiness. Depression is a factor, but daytime drowsiness occurs in people who are not depressed. Between 1918 and 1926, an epidemic of encephalitis swept the world, affecting 15 million people. The encephalitis was called "sleeping sickness" because people affected slept during the day and were awake at night. Among the people who survived, 40% had daytime drowsiness, 40% developed PD, and many people had both. Because the centers that regulate sleep are near the substantia nigra, this becomes understandable and may explain why PD and the treatment for PD may cause drowsiness.

A separate issue is whether agonists cause sleep attacks — sudden episodes of falling asleep without warning, without being drowsy. When studied in a sleep laboratory, it is found among people on agonists that sleep attacks are rare and unusual episodes. The overwhelming number of episodes that were said to be sleep attacks were episodes of falling asleep without remembering you were drowsy. If you are taking a dopamine agonist and are drowsy you should not drive.

What Agonists Are Available?

Since 1970, shortly after Sinemet was introduced, several agonists were developed. The following are currently available Apomorphine, Cabergoline, Lisuride, Mirapex (pramipexole), Parlodel (bromocriptine), Permax (pergolide), and Requip (ropinerole). Several other agonists (including one given through a patch) are being studied. The agonists below are, at present, the most effective and widely used.

Mirapex, Permax, and Requip — each is an effective drug. Each can be used alone, as initial treatment in PD. Used alone each is almost as potent as Sinemet. And almost 50% of people with PD can be maintained on each agonist for several years without Sinemet or with little Sinemet. The other 50% require almost full supplementation with Sinemet or Sinemet plus Comtan. The advantages of Mirapex, Permax, or Requip as a sole agent, or combined with Sinemet plus Comtan is that people have fewer on-off or dyskinesias. The disadvantages of Mirapex, Permax, or Requip are the slow build-up period and the higher number of hallucinations. Mirapex, Permax, and Requip can also be combined with Sinemet plus Comtan in people who are already having on-off or dyskinesias. If Sinemet can be reduced, adding Mirapex, Permax, or Requip, reduces dyskinesias. Mirapex, Permax, and Requip have increased the range of options available to people with PD. Used alone or combined with Sinemet or Sinemet plus Comtan, they have prolonged the period of time in which you can be effectively treated, and have improved the quality of life of many people.

Mirapex

Dosage forms: 0.125 mg, 0.25 mg, 1 mg, and 1.5 mg tablets
Usual daily dose: 1.5 to 4.5 mg, usually given three times per day.
Half-life: Approximately 8 hours.

Mirapex is not metabolized in the liver, but is excreted in the kidney. This may circumvent interactions with other drugs that are metabolized in the liver. Mirapex stimulates the D-3 receptor and this may account, in part, for the ability of Mirapex in some people to reduce anxiety or depression.

Common side effects: dizziness on standing, drowsiness, nausea. These can be overcome by a slow buildup. If nausea is a problem see pg. 233. If drowsiness is a problem this may be overcome by not exceeding 1.5 mg (total) per day. Swelling of the legs occurs in about 10% of people. This can be overcome by reducing the dose of Mirapex or by daily exercise, such as riding a stationery bicycle for 30 minutes. Diuretics (water pills) are usually not helpful. Hallucinations occur in older people or in those with a decline in intellect. In this instance Mirapex should be reduced or stopped.

Permax

Dosage form: 0.05, 0.25, and 1 mg tablets
Usual daily dose: 0.75 to 5.0 mg daily, usually given three times per day

Permax is metabolized in the liver and excreted by the kidneys. Of the three agonists, Permax is the only one that stimulates, in part, the D-1 receptor.

Common side effects: dizziness on standing, drowsiness, nausea. These can be overcome by a slow build-up. If nausea is a problem see how this can be overcome by reading pages 232–234. If drowsiness is a problem, this may be overcome by reducing the dose. Swelling of the legs can be overcome by reducing the dose, or by daily exercise. Hallucinations occur in older people or people with a decline in intellect. In this instance Permax should be reduced or stopped.

Requip

Dosage forms: 0.25 mg, 0.5 mg, 1 mg, 2 mg, and 5 mg tablets
Usual daily dose: 0.75 to 24 mg, given three times per day
Half-life: about 8 hours.

Requip is metabolized in the liver, and is excreted in the kidney. One of the metabolites of Requip is also effective. In some people this may be an advantage.

Common side effects: dizziness on standing, drowsiness, and nausea. These can be overcome by a slow build-up. If nausea is a problem see pages 232–234. If drowsiness is a problem this may be overcome by reducing the dose. Swelling of the legs can be overcome by reducing the dose or by daily exercise. Hallucinations occur in older people or those with a decline in intellect. In this instance, Requip should be reduced or stopped.

Nausea in Parkinson Disease

PD drugs such as Sinemet or Sinemet plus Comtan or dopamine agonists are the most frequent cause of nausea in PD. However, nausea may also occur in people not taking any PD drug. In one study, 15% of people with PD not taking PD drugs had nausea and 40% complained of abdominal fullness. Attempts to explain this focus on the stomach. The stomach normally empties its contents after the contents have been mixed and digested by stomach acid. If, as in PD, the stomach doesn't empty fully or quickly, the contents accumulate. This can result in nausea, abdominal discomfort, fullness, and even vomiting.

To reach the bloodstream (and ultimately the brain), Sinemet must pass through the stomach intact and then be absorbed in the small intestine. If Sinemet is trapped in the stomach several things happen. While trapped in the stomach, enzymes change Sinemet to dopamine, which means Sinemet can't be absorbed in the small intestine. To make matters worse, the dopamine formed in the stomach can stimulate dopamine receptors in the stomach, further delaying emptying.

If this is happening in your stomach, you may get little benefit from Sinemet, and the accumulated dopamine may make you nauseated. Some doctors feel this accounts for some (though not all) of the unpredictability of responsiveness to Sinemet.

If nausea occurs with Sinemet, this may indicate Sinemet is trapped in your stomach and that the dopa decarboxylase in your stomach is changing levodopa to dopamine. The dopamine, in turn, causes nausea. The nausea of the dopamine agonists may be different. Not only may the agonists stimulate dopamine receptors in the stomach, they may also stimulate dopamine receptors in the vomiting center of the brain.

For the nausea of Sinemet, or Sinemet plus Comtan, add carbidopa, the carbidopa of the levodopa in Sinemet. This can be prescribed by your doctor and is available as Lodosyn. The exact amount of carbidopa necessary to block the dopa decarboxylase in the stomach, liver, kidney, and blood vessels is at least 75 mg per day. It may be higher in some people. If you're nauseated on Sinemet, or Sinemet plus Comtan, add Lodosyn 25 mg to each dose of Sinemet. If after a week you are still nauseated add 50 mg of carbidopa to each dose of Sinemet. If the nausea continues you must look into other causes of nausea such as an ulcer in your stomach or your small intestine, or liver or gall bladder disease.

If you're nauseated on a dopamine agonist, or if you're nauseated on Sinemet despite adding Lodosyn, ask your doctor about prescribing Motilium (domperidone). Domperidone is a dopamine antagonist and blocks the dopamine receptors in your stomach, overcoming the nausea of dopamine agonists or Sinemet. The dose is 10 mg, three times a day. Because domperidone does not get into the brain, it cannot, like other antagonists, block the dopamine receptors in the brain. Domperidone is not available in the United

States, but information on how to obtain it, easily and legally, can be obtained by going to www.parkinson.org.

Dyskinesias

Dyskinesias occur in people with PD. They are related to the underlying disease and to the effects of Sinemet. They occur on agonists but much less frequently. In many people dyskinesias limit treatment. They usually occur in association with on-off, but the mechanisms in the brain responsible for dyskinesias is probably different.

Dyskinesia Self-evaluation Form

If you have dyskinesias, writhing or wiggling movements, learn to evaluate them. It can help in managing your PD. It can help in adjusting your drugs. It can help in determining if you might benefit from deep brain stimulation (DBS). Evaluate your dyskinesias 30 minutes after you take your first, second, third, or fourth dose of Sinemet (carbidopa/levodopa). Determine which dose of carbidopa/levodopa, the first, second, third, or fourth, results in the most dyskinesias. If the first dose (or the second dose, etc.) of carbidopa/levodopa results in the most dyskinesias, evaluate your dyskinesias after your first dose (or your second dose, etc.) of carbidopa/levodopa. Keep these records for your doctor. Dyskinesias are related to the timing of your carbidopa/levodopa. To obtain a score for dyskinesias you must know the following:

1. **Frequency**
   0: None, dyskinesias do not occur with any dose of carbidopa/levodopa. 2: Dyskinesias occur once per day after one dose of carbidopa/levodopa, but not after any other dose. 3: Dyskinesias occur twice or more times per day, but not after each dose of carbidopa/levodopa. 4: Dyskinesias occur after each dose of carbidopa/levodopa.

DYSKINESIA QUESTIONNAIRE

Left Side of Body:
Arm and/or Leg

Frequency

- ❑ 0: NONE
- ❑ 2: Once per day
- ❑ 3: More than once per day, BUT not with each dose of carbidopa/levodopa
- ❑ 4: With each dose of carbidopa/levodopa

Duration
Rate the Longest Episode

- ❑ 0: NONE
- ❑ 2: Less than 5 minutes
- ❑ 3: 5 minutes to one hour
- ❑ 4: More than one hour

Severity
Rate the most severe episode, the episode of greatest amplitude

- ❑ 0: NONE
- ❑ 2: Barely visible
- ❑ 3: Visibile, does not interfere with actions of arm or leg
- ❑ 4: Visible, interferes with actions of arm or leg

TOTAL Left Side __________

Right Side of Body:
Arm and/or Leg

Frequency

- ❑ 0: NONE
- ❑ 2: Once per day
- ❑ 3: More than once per day, BUT not with each dose of carbidopa/levodopa
- ❑ 4: With each dose of carbidopa/levodopa

Duration
Rate the Longest Episode

- ❑ 0: NONE
- ❑ 2: Less than 5 minutes
- ❑ 3: 5 minutes to one hour
- ❑ 4: More than one hour

Severity
Rate the most severe episode, the episode of greatest amplitude

- ❑ 0: NONE
- ❑ 2: Barely visible
- ❑ 3: Visibile, does not interfere with actions of arm or leg
- ❑ 4: Visible, interferes with actions of arm or leg

TOTAL Right Side __________

Results of Evaluation

TOTAL Right Side + Left Side: _______

2. **Duration**
   0: None, dyskinesias do not occur with any dose of carbidopa/levodopa. 2: The longest episode of dyskinesias lasts less than 5 minutes. 3: The longest episode lasts from 5 minutes to one hour. 4: The longest episode lasts more than one hour.
3. **Severity Rate the severity in either the arm or the leg, the limb in which the amplitude of the dyskinesias is greatest.**
   0: None. 2: Dyskinesias are barely visible. 3: Dyskinesias are visible but do not interfere with action of the arm or the leg. 4: Dyskinesias are visible AND interfere with action of the arm or the leg.

The questionnaire on page 235 is designed to help the Parkinson patient keep track of the progress of his/her disease. This questionnaire has not been scientifically validated; it is meant for educational purposes to give people with PD an understanding of how dyskinesias are evaluated.

Trihexyphenidyl

Brand name: Artane
Dosage forms: 2 mg and 5 mg immediate-release tablets; 5 mg sustained-release capsules
Usual daily dose: 2 to 10 mg in three divided dosages
Side effects: dry mouth, constipation, nausea, vomiting, blurred vision, urinary hesitancy, impaired memory, confusion, and difficulty swallowing or speaking
Drug interactions: The following drugs should be taken with caution if you are taking trihexyphenidyl:
amantadine (Symmetrel)
digoxin (Lanoxin)

Benztropine

Brand name: Cogentin
Dosage forms: 0.5 mg, 2 mg, and 5 mg tablets
Usual daily dose: 0.5 to 6 mg, two to four times per day
Side effects: dry mouth, constipation, nausea, vomiting, blurred vision, urinary hesitancy, impaired memory, confusion, and difficulty swallowing or speaking
Drug interactions: The following drugs should be taken with caution if you are taking benztropine:
amantadine (Symmetrel)
digoxin (Lanoxin)

Amantadine

Brand name: Symmetrel
Dosage forms: 100 mg capsules; syrup
Usual daily dose: 100 mg twice daily up to as much as 200 mg twice daily (total dose 400 mg per day)
Side effects: swelling of the feet, dizziness, loss of appetite, hallucinations, and blotchy skin on the legs
Drug interactions: The following drugs should be taken with caution if you are taking amantadine:
anticholinergic drugs (because amantadine has its own anticholinergic effect)

Surgery for Parkinson Disease

Initially, medication, such as levodopa/carbidopa (Sinemet, Atamet) or dopamine agonists (Mirapex, Permax, Requip) help people with PD, but eventually patients lose their benefit or develop side effects — principally dykinesias. Some patients who lose their benefit or develop dyskinesias may benefit from surgery. It is important to note that surgery isn't a cure and that patients who never responded or responded poorly to levodopa/carbidopa may not be helped by surgery.

History of Surgery in Parkinson

Surgery for Parkinson disease and other movement disorders was pioneered in the 1940s by Russel Meyers. Large regions of the brain were exposed and using surface landmarks (there were no CT-scans or MRIs), the basal ganglia — a series of interconnected regions of the brain including the striatum, globus pallidus, and thalamus, were located and destroyed. E. A. Spiegel and H. T Wycis in 1947 developed a crown-like stereotaxic frame that held the head in place and allowed regions inside the brain to be correlated with reference points on the frame. In the 1950s, Lars Leksell (Sweden) pioneered pallidotomy for tremor. Later, in the late 1950s and 1960s, Irving Cooper (United States) and Hiero Narabayashi (Japan) pioneered thalamotomy for tremor. The introduction of levodopa dramatically reduced the need for surgery. Laurie Laitinen (Sweden) and Mahlor De Long (United States), however, revived surgery by demonstrating the effectiveness of pallidotomy for levodopa-induced dyskinesias. Alim Louis Benebid (France) pioneered deep brain stimulation (DBS) of the subthalamic - nucleus (STN). A. Lozano (Canada), Anthony Lang (Canada), and William Koller (United States) refined DBS for PD and Essential Tremor. All of these pioneers dramatically increased our understanding of the brain's anatomy, circuitry, and its effects on movement.

Currently three types of surgery are performed:

1. Ablative or destructive surgery
2. Stimulatıon surgery or deep brain stimulation (DBS)
3. Transplantation or restorative surgery

Ablative or destructive surgery refers to locating, targeting, and then ablating or destroying a specific, clearly defined brain region a region that's been altered or changed by PD, a region that generates or produces an abnormal chemical or electrical discharge, an abnormal discharge that, in turn, generates an abnormal signal or "static." The static, in turn, interrupts the normal, harmonious operation of the brain. Destruction of the abnormal region lessens the static. This allows restoration of normal or closer to normal function. Destruction of the abnormal region rarely results in restoration of normal function.

A frequently asked question is "Why doesn't destruction of the abnormal region restore normal function?" The brain is more than a circuit board. There's more wrong in PD than one abnormal region. Only part of the abnormal region may have been destroyed and, at a later date, the surgeon may have to operate again. To understand why only part of the abnormal region may be destroyed requires more understanding of the surgery.

To destroy the abnormal region, the surgeon heats the exploring probe or electrode — this coagulates or destroys the abnormal region. Because the patient is awake during surgery, the surgeon can monitor the extent of the destruction by observing the patient. As an example, a patient with a left-hand tremor has the probe inserted into his brain's right side. The brain's right side controls the body's left side and vice versa. The surgeon then coagulates part of the patient's right thalamus, the abnormal region. The abnormal electrical discharge is monitored through the probe. When the patient's tremor ceases the probe is removed.

Heating causes the surrounding thalamus to swell. Initially, the swelling inactivates a wider region than is required to stop the tremor. After several weeks, the swelling subsides. Part of the thalamus remains quiet — no longer discharging. But part may recover — and the tremor may return. For example, if you burn your hand — the equivalent of heating the thalamus — the swelling of your hand peaks in 48 hours, then subsides. The full extent of the burn, won't be known for days until the swelling subsides. Few surgeons can correctly estimate the size of the burn needed to permanently abolish a tremor. It is safer to destroy a smaller region and chance the tremor returning, then to destroy a larger region and risk paralysis.

The surgery, ablative surgery and DBS, is painless. The scalp, which contains pain-sensitive nerves, is numbed with a local anesthetic. Next, a small hole is drilled into the skull. The underlying brain-covering, the dura, contains pain-sensitive nerves; they too are numbed with a local anesthetic. The brain itself contains no pain-sensitive nerves and feels no pain. Thus surgery on the brain is painless.

Ablative surgery doesn't cure PD; a troubling symptom may be abolished, but PD is not. PD is a progressive disease — other symptoms eventually appear.

Deep brain stimulation, DBS, refers to implanting a probe or electrode into a clearly defined, abnormal brain region, a region generating "static." This is usually, but not always, the same region targeted in destructive surgery. By generating a blocking counter-current the effects of the static are negated. Technically, DBS is a misnomer — the abnormal discharging brain region isn't stimulated — it's blocked by a reverse or counter-current.

Destructive surgery targets the globus pallidus or thalamus. The words for this surgery are pallodotomy and thalamotomy. *Pallidotomy* means literally putting a "hole" or an "otomy" into the globus pallidus. *Thalamotomy* means putting a "hole" or an "otomy" into the thalamus.

DBS targets the globus pallidus, or thalamus or subthalamic nucleus (STN). The STN is below the thalamus. The STN is a small region harder to target than the globus pallidus or thalamus. In a person without PD, destruction of one STN, by a stroke or tumor, results in uncontrolled, involuntary movements on the opposite side of the body. These movements are a form of dyskinesia. In a person with PD, destruction of one STN by a stroke, results in restoration of near normal movement on the opposite side. This observation formed the basis for DBS of the STN. DBS is chosen over destruction of the STN because the resulting inactivation of the STN can be more accurately and precisely regulated — and, if necessary, reversed. Few people are willing to risk the possibility that destruction of the STN might result in dyskinesias.

Advantages of DBS over Destructive Surgery

With DBS the targeted region is preserved not destroyed. If necessary, inactivation of the target can be reversed by turning off the current.

With DBS a more accurate and precise control of symptoms is possible.

There is a greater risk of hemorrhage or stroke with destructive surgery than with DBS.

Disadvantages of DBS over Destructive Surgery

The patient has an implanted electrode in his brain. This can become infected.

The electrode is connected through a wire running down the patient's neck, under his skin, to a stimulator and battery-pack under the chest wall (similar to a cardiac pacemaker).

The stimulator is turned on or off with an external magnet. The wire from the brain to the chest can become infected — or break. The battery must be replaced, through a minor surgical incision, every three to five years (similar to a pacemaker).

The stimulator may have to be periodically reprogrammed. This requires a level of expertise not universally available. While it is an annoyance, it is better than having a surgeon go back inside the brain and perform another destructive lesion.

For most patients DBS is a better choice than ablative or destructive surgery.

Some frequently asked questions are:

1. How safe are the procedures?
2. Is there more risk in destructive surgery than in DBS?
3. Who pays for the procedure?

The answers are as follows:

1. Every surgical procedure carries a risk; it is naive to think otherwise. The surgery is done because the patient, his doctor, and the surgeon concluded the benefit of the surgery, abolition of tremor, abolition of dyskinesia, or restoration of movement outweighed the risk and a comparable result could not be achieved with medicines. The risks of any procedure are higher in older people, more debilitated people, people with cerebral atrophy (shrinkage of

brain tissue as documented by CAT scans, or MRIs), and people with additional conditions, such as high blood pressure, bleeding or clotting tendencies, heart disease, or seizures. None of the preceding conditions are "no-no's" — they entail more discussion, more thought, and more precautions.

The major risks in the surgery are the risks of inserting a hard metallic probe or electrode past the surface of the brain and guiding the probe to the target.

One risk is hemorrhage or bleeding. The brain is richly covered with blood vessels — large and small. The surgery may be contraindicated or special precautions may have to be taken in people with a tendency to bleed, such as in people on drugs such as aspirin or coumadin. Recommendations regarding the length of time people should discontinue aspirin or coumadin before surgery vary. Bleeding inside the brain may be minor and without consequences, or it may be major, resulting in paralysis or death.

A second risk is stroke. The stroke may be minor with full recovery, or it may be major — with partial or complete permanent paralysis of an arm and/or a leg.

The combined risk of bleeding or stroke resulting in serious disability, is one to three percent at hospitals with excellent reputations and experience in selecting patients and performing the surgery.

A third risk is infection. There are several other risks, detailed on the operative consent form. The patient, his spouse, and family should ask to see a copy of this before entering the hospital, while they are at home and can study them at leisure. Everyone, patient, spouse, and concerned family members should understand the potential benefits and risks.

2. There's a risk of hemorrhage or stroke with destructive surgery and DBS. The risk occurs when the brain is penetrated by the probe or electrode. With destructive surgery there is an added risk as the targeted region is coagulated. How much added risk? The answer varies depending on the patient, the procedure, and the surgeon. Patients with a bleeding tendency, uncontrolled high-blood pressure, or with cerebral atrophy are more at risk for bleeding with any surgical procedure. However, they are more at risk for bleeding with destructive surgery than DBS.
3. Payments vary from state to state, from insurance company to insurance company, and from surgery to surgery. The government, Medicare, which will pay for a procedure in one state will refuse to pay in another state. Before scheduling surgery check with your insurance carrier and, preferably, have a commitment in writing beforehand.

The Globus Pallidus and Its Connections

The globus pallidus is a pale, globe-like region deep inside the brain situated below the striatum and above the substantia nigra. The substantia nigra is a darkly pigmented region, hence its name from the Latin, dark (nigra) substance. The substantia nigra contains approximately 400,000 dopamine producing nerve cells, 200,000 on each side. The entire brain contains 10 billion nerve cells. Thus the substantia nigra represents only 0.004% of the brain's nerve cells. But what an important number! When a person loses 240,000 nerve cells, 60% of the nerve cells in the substantia nigra — he develops the first symptoms of PD. When a person loses 360,000 nerve cells, 90% of the nerve cells in the substantia nigra — he has advanced PD.

The dopamine-producing cells in the substantia nigra project to nerve cells in the striatum. The connections are made on specialized places, receptors on nerve cells in the striatum. These are the dopamine receptors. They are proteins upon which levodopa and the dopamine agonists — Mirapex, Permax, and Requip— act. In addition to nerve cells from the substantia nigra, the striatum also receives nerve cells from the cerebral cortex. One group of nerve cells in the striatum project to the inner part of the globus pallidus. Here information on movement, balance, and posture is exchanged, analyzed, interpreted, and integrated with information from other brain regions.

A second group of nerve cells projects from the striatum first to a group of nerve cells in the outer segment of the globus pallidus. Here information is exchanged, analyzed, interpreted, and integrated with additional information from other brain regions. Then the nerve cells in the outer segment of the globus pallidus project to the STN. Here information is again exchanged, analyzed, interpreted, and integrated with additional information from other brain regions. Next, the nerve cells in the STN project to the inner part segment of the globus pallidus. Here information is exchanged, analyzed, interpreted, and integrated with additional information from other brain regions.

In PD, the inner part of the globus pallidus becomes "over" active and generates "static." Creating a small hole in the internal globus pallidus, or inserting a probe and generating a countercurrent (as in DBS), decreases the amount of abnormal signals originating from the innner part of the globus pallidus. This in turn normalizes or calms the electrical activity in a larger brain circuit.

Explaining the actions of the globus pallidus requires using an analogy. In PD, as the substantia nigra nerve cells die and movement slows down, picture a car running out of gas. The globus pallidus, which normally functions as a brake, is, paradoxically, turned on, resulting in further slowing of movement. DBS of the globus pallidus is equivalent to releasing a brake — and increasing movement. This analogy doesn't explain how DBS decreases dyskinesias or tremor. That DBS can increase movement and decrease dyskinesias and tremor implies that the mechanism underlying normal movement and excessive movement are different. This is under investigation.

The inner part of the globus pallidus is organized segmentally: there's a part for the head, a part for the trunk, a part for the arm and leg. The globus pallidus on the brain's right side controls the body's left side. However, there's overlap; the right globus pallidus affects, partly, the body's right side, and vice versa. Often, DBS on one side decreases dyskinesias or improves movement of both sides of the body. The inner part of the globus pallidus, in addition to receiving information on movement, receives information from regions of the brain that regulate emotions. Facetiously, the activity of the globus pallidus may be summarized in terms such as "jumping for joy" or "hopping mad."

The nerve cells in the inner part of the globus pallidus are electrically and chemically distinct from the nerve cells in the outer part of the globus pallidus. The nerve cells in the inner part of the globus pallidus have a characteristic of discharge or fire and emit a high-pitched sound. The nerve cells in the outer part of the globus pallidus emit a low-pitched sound. The sounds can be listened to through the probe and displayed on an oscilloscope. This is called micro electrode recording. The sounds are as distinctive, one from the other, as a radio station playing rock-and-roll is from a station playing classical music.

Micro electrode recording is supplemented with macro electrode stimulation. Macro electrode stimulation refers to applying an electrical current to a region of the brain and observing its effect, for example noting if it results in movement of an arm versus a leg. Micro electrode recording and macro electrode stimulation are checks on location. Thus a region of the brain, the globus pallidus or thalamus, is located by MRI-guidance — much the way a pilot locates a village or town from an airplane. Micro electrode recording and macro electrode stimulation allow the pilot to confirm his location by listening to local chatter.

Micro electrode recording increases the length of surgery. Some surgeons say micro electrode recording increases the risk of surgery: the more you probe and listen — the higher the risk of bleeding. Most surgeons, however, use micro electrode recording in addition to MRI-localization, because micro electrode recording provides a degree of precision and accuracy not possible with MRI alone. The surgeons who don't use micro electrode recordings rely on MRI-localization supplemented by macro electrode stimulation.

The inner part of the globus pallidus projects to the thalamus. The thalamus is a major relay station in the brain. The thalamus receives information on sensation: touch, hot and cold, pressure, and pain. The thalamus exchanges, analyzes, interprets, and integrates this information with information from the globus pallidus, the cerebellum (a region that regulates balance), and other regions and relays this information to the cerebral cortex — the thinking part of the brain. The thalamus is organized regionally: there's a part for pain sensation, a part for movement, a part for balance. The thalamus on the brain's right side controls the body's left side and vice versa.

Since the thalamus receives a major input from the globus pallidus, one would expect destruction of the thalamus and of the globus pallidus to be equivalent. They're not. Destruction (thalamotomy), or DBS of the thalamus results in lessening of tremor — on the opposite side of the body. Thalamotomy or DBS of the thalamus doesn't lessen dyskinesias and doesn't improve movement. Most surgeons prefer thalamotomy or DBS of the thalamus over pallidototomy or DBS of the pallidus as a treatment for tremor — where tremor, not slowed movement, is the major problem. Reasons given include that the thalamus is easier to target than the globus pallidus; not everyone agrees.

In people with Essential Tremor, a condition in which the tremor is present only when the hand contracts or moves, DBS is preferred over thalamotomy.

The Subthalamic Nucleus, STN

The STN is a small region below the thalamus. Today, many researchers consider the STN to have a role in PD comparable in magnitude, but opposite in direction, to the substantia nigra. As the substantia nigra "turns-off," the STN "turns-on."

Inactivating the STN with DBS has, in some patients, an effect comparable to levodopa; so dramatic an effect that many surgeons consider DBS of the STN superior to DBS of the globus pallidus. Some surgeons disagree. A study comparing the efficacy and safety of DBS of the STN with DBS of the globus pallidus will soon commence. Until the study is completed and the data analyzed people must rely on the opinion of their surgeon.

Procedures on Both Sides (Bilateral) Versus Procedures on One Side (Unilateral)

PD is usually asymmetrical, that is, one side is affected more than the other. Thus, tremor is usually worse in one hand than the other, dyskinesias are usually more pronounced on one side than the other. In such people, one-sided thalamotomy or pallidotomy or one-sided DBS of the thalamus, globus pallidus, or STN is enough. Some people, however, require a second operation. There may be "hidden" risks in the second operation. Functions such as intelligence, speech, and balance are represented bilaterally in the brain. The small and appropriately placed "holes" made on one side of the brain during pallidotomy or thalamotomy usually don't affect intelligence, speech, or balance. However, in some people, perhaps 5% (higher in patients with a history of mini-strokes or confusion), a second small and appropriately placed "hole" made on the other side of the brain can affect intelligence, speech, or balance. It is especially so when the "holes" are made during the same operation; it is less likely when the "holes" are made during separate operations — several weeks or months apart. The exact reason for this is unknown. It is theorized that the brain has a certain resilience. This "resilience" allows the brain to compensate for a single "hole" on one side by shifting functions such as intelligence, speech, and balance to the other side. Now, a second "hole" on the opposite side has an unexpected effect.

If people require bilateral operations the surgeon can do a thalamotomy or pallidotomy on one side followed by DBS of the other side. Or the surgeon can do DBS on both sides. This is another advantage of DBS. DBS of both sides (thalamus, globus pallidus,

STN) is usually safer than thalamotomy or pallidotomy of both sides.

Transplantation

Transplantation surgery transfers or implants, dopamine-producing cells into the striatum. Cells are transplanted into the striatum because it is easier and safer to locate and target than the smaller and less accessible substantia nigra. Because the foreign cells aren't transplanted into the nigra they can't exactly replicate the lost nigral cells. As an example, dopamine cells in the nigra receive, exchange, analyze, and interpret information from other brain regions including cells in the brainstem (a region below the nigra). Dopamine cells transplanted into the striatum don't receive, exchange, analyze, and interpret information from the brainstem.

Transplanted cells can come from several sources. Once implanted, the cells then attempt to compensate for the lost cells in the patient's substantia nigra. There are 400,000 nerve cells in the substantia nigra, 200,000 on each side. When a person loses 240,000 cells, 60% of his total, PD first appears. This implies that 160,000 cells, 40%, is the minimum needed to maintain normal movement. Approximately 80% to 90% of transplanted cells die during implantation, failing to take hold or establish connections within the brain. Successful transplantation usually requires at least 1,600,000 cells, 10 times the minimum. If human embryos are used, transplantation requires at least three to four embryos with 400,000 cells in each embryo.

Transplantation surgery seeks to re-establish dopamine levels in the brain while setting back the "PD clock" — returning the patient to a less advanced disease stage. Transplantation is usually performed bilaterally. In some hospitals surgery is performed on both sides at the same setting. In other hospitals surgery is performed in stages: first one side, then several weeks or months later, the other side. The surgery is performed stereotaxically — with the patient asleep. The surgery carries approximately the same risk as destructive surgery: a one to three percent risk of hemorrhage, stroke, or death. Unlike destructive surgery or DBS, the benefits of transplantation are not apparent for months — because the transplanted cells must integrate themselves into the person's brain.

Most, but not all, people who undergo transplantation surgery are treated with immunosuppressive drugs to prevent the brain from rejecting the cells. There's a difference of opinion among researchers as to the necessity of using immunosuppressive drugs.

Sources of transplanted cells include:

Cells from the patient's adrenal gland. These cells resemble but are not identical to dopamine-producing cells. This approach was pioneered by I. Madrazo (Mexico). It was successful in few patients. Most PD patients had difficulty undergoing simultaneous operations: one on their belly to remove their adrenal gland, then one on their brain to implant the adrenal gland. The survival rate of adrenal tissue in the brain is poor. This approach has been abandoned.

Cells from the patient's carotid body. A small cluster of dopamine-producing cells encircle the carotid artery in the neck. These cells are removed and implanted into the person's brain. This operation has had limited success — probably because there aren't enough cells to implant in the brain.

Cells from aborted human embryos. Anders Bjorkland and Ollie Lindvall (Sweden) pioneered this approach and much of our knowledge of human transplantation. The social and ethical concerns surrounding the use of human embryos, the difficulty of obtaining an adequate number of embryos, and the dissimilarity among embryos has limited this surgery.

The embryonic tissue is usually transplanted into the putamen, part of the striatum. The putamen is involved in directing and regulating movement. In time, after several months, the transplanted tissue integrates itself into the brain and acts as a pump injecting dopamine directly into the putamen.

A recent study conducted in a randomized, double-blind manner including "sham" surgery demonstrated transplantation is beneficial in only some patients — predominantly those less than 60 years. About 15% of people developed dyskinesias. This procedure has largely been abandoned.

- *Cells from pig embryos.* Pigs are, immunologically, close to humans. An unlimited number, millions and millions of cells, from specifically bred, developed, and prepared pig embryos can be made available for transplantation.

How many people have surgery? It is estimated there are 1,000,000 PD patients in the United States. Fewer than 1,000 patients, less than 0.1% of PD patients, undergo surgery each year. Why so few? The surgery isn't for newly diagnosed people; people doing well on medication; people with advanced disease who aren't responding to medication; people with hallucinations, confusion, or memory loss; or people who are or afraid.

How many people are candidates for surgery? Perhaps (my estimate) 10% of PD people are candidates for surgery. As surgery is improved and perfected, as it becomes safer, as new techniques and strategies are innovated, developed, and applied — a larger number of people will opt for and benefit from surgery.

A new and promising approach is gene therapy. This has been successfully performed in monkeys in one approach, by Dr. Krys Bankiewicz, the gene for making dopamine is inserted into the striatum. This converts the striatal cells that are normal into dopamine factories. In a second approach, by Dr. Jeff Kordover, a gene for repairing dopamine cells is inserted into the substantia nigra or the striatum.